PSYCHOPHARMACOLOGICAL TREATMENT COMPLICATIONS IN THE ELDERLY

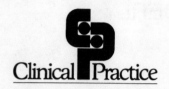

Clinical Practice

Number 23
Judith H. Gold, M.D., F.R.C.P.(C)
Series Editor

PSYCHOPHARMACOLOGICAL TREATMENT COMPLICATIONS IN THE ELDERLY

Edited by

Charles A. Shamoian, M.D., Ph.D.

Professor of Clinical Psychiatry
Cornell University Medical College
New York, New York

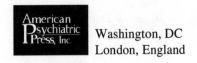
Washington, DC
London, England

Note: The authors have worked to ensure that all information in this book concerning drug dosages, schedules, and routes of administration is accurate as of the time of publication and consistent with standards set by the U.S. Food and Drug Administration and the general medical community. As medical research and practice advance, however, therapeutic standards may change. For this reason and because human and mechanical errors sometimes occur, we recommend that readers follow the advice of a physician who is directly involved in their care or the care of a member of their family.

Books published by the American Psychiatric Press, Inc., represent the views and opinions of the individual authors and do not necessarily represent the policies and opinions of the Press or the American Psychiatric Association.

Copyright © 1992 American Psychiatric Press, Inc.
ALL RIGHTS RESERVED
Manufactured in the United States of America on acid-free paper.
First Edition   93 92 91 4 3 2 1

American Psychiatric Press, Inc.
1400 K Street, N.W., Washington, DC 20005

Library of Congress Cataloging-in-Publication Data

Psychopharmacological treatment complications in the elderly /
    edited by Charles A. Shamoian. — 1st ed.
    p. cm. — (Clinical practice : no. 23)
    Consists of updated and revised papers presented at a symposium
held at the Annual Meeting of the American Psychiatric
Association, San Francisco, 1989.
    Includes bibliographical references.
    ISBN 0-88048-459-4 (alk. paper)
    1. Geriatric pharmacology—Congresses. 2. Psychotropic drugs—
Side effects—Congresses. I. Shamoian, Charles A., 1931–   . II.
American Psychiatric Association. Meeting (142nd : 1989 : San
Francisco, Calif.). III. Series.
    [DNLM: 1. Mental Disorders—drug therapy—congresses. 2.
Mental Disorders—in old age—congresses. 3. Psychotropic Drugs—
adverse effects—congresses.   W1 CL767J no. 23 / QV 77 P97205
1989]
RC953.7.P77 1991
615'. 78—dc20
DNLM/DLC   91-25951
for Library of Congress   CIP

British Library Cataloguing in Publication Data

A CIP record is available from the British Library.

Contents

Contributors

Gerard Addonizio, M.D.
Associate Professor of Clinical Psychiatry
Cornell University Medical College
New York, New York

Michel Calache, M.D.
Fellow in Geriatric Psychiatry
Southern Illinois University School of Medicine
Springfield, Illinois

Vinod Kumar, M.D., M.R.C.Psych.
Associate Professor of Psychiatry
Southern Illinois University School of Medicine
Springfield, Illinois

Barnett S. Meyers, M.D.
Associate Professor of Clinical Psychiatry
Cornell University Medical College
New York, New York

M. Michele Murburg, M.D.
Assistant Professor of Psychiatry
University of Washington School of Medicine
Seattle, Washington

Marcella Pascualy, M.D.
Acting Instructor in Psychiatry
University of Washington School of Medicine
Seattle, Washington

Charles A. Shamoian, M.D., Ph.D.
Professor of Clinical Psychiatry
Cornell University Medical College
New York, New York

Javaid I. Sheikh, M.D.
Assistant Professor of Psychiatry
Stanford University Medical Center
Stanford, California

Larry E. Tune, M.D.
Associate Professor of Psychiatry
The Johns Hopkins University School of Medicine
Baltimore, Maryland

Richard C. Veith, M.D.
Professor of Psychiatry
University of Washington School of Medicine
Seattle, Washington

Introduction
to the Clinical Practice Series

Over the years of its existence the series of monographs entitled *Clinical Insights* gradually became focused on providing current, factual, and theoretical material of interest to the clinician working outside of a hospital setting. To reflect this orientation, the name of the Series has been changed to *Clinical Practice.*

The Clinical Practice Series will provide readers with books that give the mental health clinician a practical clinical approach to a variety of psychiatric problems. These books will provide up-to-date literature reviews and emphasize the most recent treatment methods. Thus, the publications in the Series will interest clinicians working both in psychiatry and in the other mental health professions.

Each year a number of books will be published dealing with all aspects of clinical practice. In addition, from time to time when appropriate, the publications may be revised and updated. Thus, the Series will provide quick access to relevant and important areas of psychiatric practice. Some books in the Series will be authored by a person considered to be an expert in that particular area; others will be edited by such an expert who will also draw together other knowledgeable authors to produce a comprehensive overview of that topic.

Some of the books in the Clinical Practice Series will have their foundation in presentations at an annual meeting of the American Psychiatric Association. All will contain the most recently available information on the subjects discussed. Theoretical and scientific data will be applied to clinical situations, and case illustrations will be utilized in order to make the material even more relevant for the practitioner. Thus, the Clinical Practice Series should provide educational reading in a compact format especially written for the mental health clinician–psychiatrist.

Judith H. Gold, M.D., F.R.C.P.(C)
Series Editor
Clinical Practice Series

Clinical Practice Series Titles

Treating Chronically Mentally Ill Women (#1)
Edited by Leona L. Bachrach, Ph.D., and Carol C. Nadelson, M.D.

Divorce as a Developmental Process (#2)
Edited by Judith H. Gold, M.D., F.R.C.P.(C)

Family Violence: Emerging Issues of a National Crisis (#3)
Edited by Leah J. Dickstein, M.D., and Carol C. Nadelson, M.D.

Anxiety and Depressive Disorders in the Medical Patient (#4)
By Leonard R. Derogatis, Ph.D., and Thomas N. Wise, M.D.

Anxiety: New Findings for the Clinician (#5)
Edited by Peter Roy-Byrne, M.D.

The Neuroleptic Malignant Syndrome and Related Conditions (#6)
By Arthur Lazarus, M.D., Stephan C. Mann, M.D., and Stanley N. Caroff, M.D.

Juvenile Homicide (#7)
Edited by Elissa P. Benedek, M.D., and Dewey G. Cornell, Ph.D.

Measuring Mental Illness: Psychometric Assessment for Clinicians (#8)
Edited by Scott Wetzler, Ph.D.

Family Involvement in Treatment of the Frail Elderly (#9)
Edited by Marion Zucker Goldstein, M.D.

Psychiatric Care of Migrants: A Clinical Guide (#10)
By Joseph Westermeyer, M.D., M.P.H., Ph.D.

Office Treatment of Schizophrenia (#11)
Edited by Mary V. Seeman, M.D., F.R.C.P.(C), and Stanley E. Greben, M.D., F.R.C.P.(C)

The Psychosocial Impact of Job Loss (#12)
By Nick Kates, M.B.B.S., F.R.C.P.(C), Barrie S. Greiff, M.D., and Duane Q. Hagen, M.D.Edited by Marion Zucker Goldstein, M.D.

New Perspectives on Narcissism (#13)
Edited by Eric M. Plakun, M.D.

Clinical Management of Gender Identity Disorders in Children and Adults (#14)
Edited by Ray Blanchard, Ph.D., and Betty W. Steiner, M.B., F.R.C.P.(C)

Family Approaches in Treatment of Eating Disorders (#15)
Edited by D. Blake Woodside, M.D., M.Sc., F.R.C.P.(C), and Lorie Shekter-Wolfson, M.S.W., C.S.W.

Adolescent Psychotherapy (#16)
Edited by Marcia Slomowitz, M.D.

Benzodiazepines in Clinical Practice: Risks and Benefits (#17)
Edited by Peter P. Roy-Byrne, M.D., and Deborah S. Cowley, M.D.

Current Treatments of Obsessive-Compulsive Disorder (#18)
Edited by Michele Tortora Pato, M.D., and Joseph Zohar, M.D.

Children and AIDS (#19)
Edited by Margaret L. Stuber, M.D.

Special Problems in Managing Eating Disorders (#20)
Edited by Joel Yager, M.D., Harry E. Gwirtsman, M.D., and Carole K. Edelstein, M.D.

Suicide and Clinical Practice (#21)
Edited by Douglas Jacobs, M.D.

Anxiety Disorders in Children and Adolescents (#22)
By Syed Arshad Husain, M.D., F.R.C.P.(C), F.R.C.Psych., and Javad Kashani, M.D.

Psychopharmacological Treatment Complications in the Elderly (#23)
Edited by Charles A. Shamoian, M.D., Ph.D.

Introduction

Since their advent, psychotropic drugs have been known to ameliorate the emotional anguish of mental illness of patients spanning the life cycle. The frequent prescribing of these medications for the elderly has been documented in a number of studies.[1] Although the elderly comprise only 12% of the general population, they consume approximately 25% of the prescribed medications.[2] These medications interact with each other as well as with drugs commonly prescribed for the multiple concomitant medical illnesses. The drug-drug interactions may result in decreased therapeutic effects or adverse side effects.[3]

As is commonly known, many of the psychotropics are associated with frequent side effects that are tolerated relatively well by the younger patient but poorly by the elderly. These side effects include, for example, dry mouth, blurred vision, constipation, and dystonic reactions. Additional factors such as polypharmacy, decreased compliance, and altered pharmacokinetics and pharmacodynamics with aging complicate treatment and therapeutic response.[3] Thus writing out specific directions and frequently monitoring the elderly patient are fundamental and essential to proper clinical care. Proper care also includes informing family members and support systems. In this context a critical role of the psychiatrist is to function as a coordinator of the numerous, disparate medical services and providers. By doing so, unwanted iatrogenic and possibly lethal effects of treatment might be avoided. An example of this would be the concomitant administration of a monoamine oxidase inhibitor and meperidine.

---

[1]Greenblatt DJ, Shader RI, Koch-Weser J: Psychotropic drug use in the Boston area: a report from the Boston Collaborative Drug Surveillance Program. Arch Gen Psychiatry 32:518–523, 1975

[2]Guttman D: A study of drug-taking behavior of older Americans, in Medication Management and Education of the Elderly. Edited by Beber CR, Lamy PP. Amsterdam, Excerpta Medica, 1978, pp 18–19

[3]Jenike MA: Geriatric Psychiatry and Psychopharmacology: A Clinical Approach. Chicago, IL, Year Book Medical, 1989

Although psychotropics may have undesired side effects, they are no different than any of the other life-sustaining pharmaceutical agents such as digitalis or calcium channel–blocking agents. None of these medications are strictly organ specific or "clean," but when used appropriately they may be life saving. Indeed the psychotropics have diminished the emotional suffering of many an elderly person and have provided the foundation for additional, happy years. However, before instituting treatment with a psychotropic, the clinician should ask, "What is the benefit-risk ratio? Are there other (i.e., nonpsychotropic) approaches that could or should be used prior to resorting to these medications?"

This monograph has its basis in a symposium presented at the annual meeting of the American Psychiatric Association in San Francisco in 1989. The chapters included are updated reviews or extended studies of those topics presented at that symposium. In the first chapter, Dr. Barnett S. Meyers reviews the fundamental question of whether or not adverse cognitive effects are associated with the use of tricyclic antidepressants in the treatment of geriatric depression. Dr. R. C. Veith and colleagues, in Chapter 2, provide a comprehensive review of cardiac risks of antidepressants in the aged. Every psychiatrist realizes the clinical importance of this issue, especially in the geriatric patient, in whom cardiovascular illnesses are probably the most commonly occurring medical problems.

In Chapter 3, Dr. L. E. Tune reviews the commonly encountered toxicities associated with neuroleptic and anticholinergic medications. The former are frequently prescribed for the psychotic elderly and may induce unwanted serious side effects that may be debilitating for the elderly. One such serious adverse reaction is the neuroleptic malignant syndrome, which until recently was not thought to occur in the elderly. Dr. G. Addonizio, in Chapter 4, clearly emphasizes the differential diagnosis, which may be complex in the aged because of the presence of other neurological illnesses.

Anxiety, and specifically chronic anxiety, occur in the elderly. In Chapter 5, Dr. J. I. Sheikh addresses the controversial issue of whether to use benzodiazepines chronically in the elderly. In addition, Dr. Sheikh highlights many of the common side effects and their deleterious impact on the daily functioning of the elderly. The last chapter focuses on a topic seldom reviewed in depth. Drs. V. Kumar and M. Calache comprehensively summarize not only the therapeutic effects but also the side effects of cholinergic drugs used in the treatment of Alzheimer's disease.

These chapters have immediate application to the common, complex clinical situations so frequently encountered in the treatment of mental illness in geriatric patients who concomitantly suffer from other medical problems. Hopefully this monograph will lead to additional readings and will provide the clinician with a higher degree of sensitivity to the issue of complications associated with psychotropic treatment in the elderly. Minimizing these unwanted side effects will lessen the burden of the mentally ill elderly patient.

Charles A. Shamoian, M.D., Ph.D.

Chapter 1

Adverse Cognitive Effects of Tricyclic Antidepressants in the Treatment of Geriatric Depression: Fact or Fiction?

Barnett S. Meyers, M.D.

*T*he efficacy of "therapeutic" concentrations of tricyclic antidepressants (TCAs) for the treatment of major depression in mixed-aged adult samples is well established (American Psychiatric Association Task Force 1985). Although few studies have assessed TCA treatment in elderly depressive patients, both nortriptyline (Åsberg et al. 1971; Georgotas et al. 1986) and desipramine (Nelson et al. 1985) appear to be effective at concentrations comparable to those used in younger adults.

Benefits of TCAs must be balanced against the risk of untoward reactions. Because these agents have potent anticholinergic activity (Snyder and Yamamura 1977), and because advanced age can increase sensitivity to anticholinergic side effects (Jenike 1985), the use of TCAs can be problematic in older patients. In this chapter the focus will be on the particular anticholinergic side effect of impaired cognitive performance. Data addressing the clinical lore that elderly patients are particularly vulnerable to developing this untoward reaction and, in its extreme form, the delirium of a central anticholinergic syndrome will be reviewed. The methodological difficulty of distinguishing cognitive side effects due to TCAs from phenomenological concomitants of depression will also be discussed. Finally, data from studies specifically measuring the cognitive effects of TCAs will be described. Material will be discussed in the context of evidence suggesting that disrupted cholinergic functioning plays a role in aging-related cognitive deficits and in those deficits associated with Alzheimer's disease.

The Role of Acetylcholine in Memory, Aging, and Alzheimer's Disease

Volunteers taking anticholinergic agents under controlled conditions experience decreased memory and orientation at low doses. These deficits progress to a full-blown central anticholinergic syndrome as high dosage is reached (Ketchum et al. 1973; Safer and Allen 1971). Similarity between the memory impairment induced by the anticholinergic drug scopolamine and deficits associated with normal aging (Drachman 1977; Drachman and Leavitt 1974) has led to the suggestion that degeneration of cholinergic neurons is responsible for age-related memory loss.

The cholinergic hypothesis (Bartus et al. 1982; Smith and Swash 1978) attributes the cognitive deficits associated with Alzheimer's disease to the degeneration of cholinergic pathways running from the nucleus basalis of Meynert to the hippocampus (Whitehouse et al. 1980). Postmortem studies in patients with Alzheimer's disease demonstrate histologic evidence of hippocampal damage (Blessed et al. 1968) and histochemical evidence of degeneration of cholinergic neurons (Davies and Maloney 1976; Perry et al. 1977). Although these studies emphasize that Alzheimer's disease patients have lower cholinergic activity than age-matched control subjects, the data also demonstrate that cholinergic activity decreases with normal aging; the lowest levels of cholinergic activity are found in patients over 70 (Davies 1978).

To summarize, studies related to the cholinergic hypothesis suggest that decrements in cholinergic function contribute to the memory deficits of normal aging; in Alzheimer's disease, the loss of cholinergic neurons is progressive and severe. These conclusions suggest that cognitive functioning in elderly depressive patients, particularly those with concurrent Alzheimer's disease, will be disrupted by the anticholinergic activity of TCAs.

Tricyclic Antidepressants and the Central Anticholinergic Syndrome

The potent affinity of TCAs for muscarinic acetylcholine receptors is well documented. The binding affinity of amitriptyline for brain receptors is only one-tenth that of atropine (Richelson 1982), but the TCA, although given orally rather than parenterally, is administered at a much higher dose. The secondary amine tricyclics, such as desipramine and nortriptyline, have profoundly less anticholinergic activity (Richelson 1982) and are effective at much lower concentrations than their tertiary amine counterparts imipramine and amitriptyline.

These pharmacological data are consistent with the conclusion that TCAs have potent anticholinergic activity, with secondary amines being less likely to disrupt this neurotransmitter system and cause anticholinergic side effects.

Cognitive Side Effects Reported in the Clinical Literature

Chart review studies report that approximately 10% (Davies et al. 1971; Livingston et al. 1983) of depressed patients treated with TCAs develop a confusional syndrome attributable to central anticholinergic toxicity. The delirium occurs more frequently in older patients; Davies et al. (1971) reported an incidence of confusional episodes in 35% of TCA-treated patients over age 40. It is of note that 30 of the 31 patients with confusion in these reports received tertiary-amine TCAs. Also, delirium occurs more frequently at high TCA blood levels, especially those over 450 ng/ml (Meador-Woodruff et al. 1988; Preskorn and Simpson 1982). Thus, the greater anticholinergic activity of tertiary-amine TCAs and aging-related pharmacokinetic changes that increase the blood levels of these TCAs for a given dose (Nies et al. 1977) partially explain the high frequency of central anticholinergic syndrome noted.

We have previously reported a much lower incidence of delirium when secondary amine TCAs are used and blood levels are monitored (Meyers and Mei-Tal 1983). Only 3 of 43 (7%) of patients over age 60 developed confusional reactions; furthermore, none of the 7 patients meeting clinical criteria for Alzheimer's disease with depression developed confusion. Reynolds and coworkers (1987) published comparable data: 32 elderly major depressive patients, including 8 with Alzheimer's disease and depression, tolerated therapeutic doses of nortriptyline without worsening of cognitive performance on the Mini-Mental State Examination (MMSE) (Folstein et al. 1975). Furthermore, Reifler and colleagues (1989) reported that 27 outpatients with Alzheimer's disease tolerated approximately 80 mg/day of imipramine and blood levels averaging over 120 ng/ml without worsening of MMSE scores. Neither study reported the occurrence of delirium in the TCA-treated subjects.

Cognitive Side Effects Induced by Scopolamine in Elderly Subjects With Alzheimer's Disease or Depression

The sensitivity of elderly patients to cognitive disturbance caused by anticholinergic drugs has been assessed by comparing subjects with Alzheimer's disease, subjects with depression, and age-matched control subjects after administration of varying doses of scopolamine (Newhouse et al. 1988; Sunderland et al. 1987). The studies demonstrate that cognitive dysfunction is apparent at a lower scopolamine dose of 0.25 mg administered intravenously in Alzheimer's disease patients compared with that of 0.5 mg in the comparison groups. Although the deficits induced by scopolamine in the Alzheimer's disease subjects were found on most test measures, Alzheimer's disease patients were most sensitive on tasks requiring effort and involving new learning. These studies did not demonstrate a similar hierarchy of scopolamine sensitivity in depressed patients. The pattern of sensitivity of depressed patients was comparable to that of the control subjects; that is, depression did not appear to specifically increase sensitivity to scopolamine on tasks involving new learning or effort. (Differences in the effects of depression and Alzheimer's disease on the components of cognitive functioning will be discussed below.)

Additional Causes of Confusion During Tricyclic Antidepressant Treatment

Cognitive disturbance during TCA treatment can be caused by factors other than anticholinergic toxicity. Aggravation of psychotic symptoms in patients with delusional depression has been associated with the use of TCAs (Nelson et al. 1979). We have suggested (Meyers and Mei-Tal 1985–1986) that the high frequency of central anticholinergic syndrome reported in the chart review studies cited above (Davies et al. 1971; Livingston et al. 1983) may result from misdiagnosing an exacerbated psychosis as a delirium. Although TCAs do have subtle, yet measurable, peripheral anticholinergic effects in vivo (Szabadi et al. 1980), the absence of peripheral evidence of anticholinergic toxicity in most cases of central anticholinergic syndrome (Davies et al. 1971; Livingston et al. 1983) and in research subjects with clear cognitive and behavioral disturbance caused by scopolamine (Sunderland et al. 1987) attests to the complexity of diagnosis.

The potent binding affinities for TCAs in other neurotransmitter systems are well documented. These agents are potent blockers of alpha$_1$-adrenergic receptors and histaminic (H$_1$) receptors in human brain (Richelson 1982). Although cognitive deficits, especially those caused by diminished arousal, could be caused by the antinoradrenergic or antihistaminic properties of these agents, TCA blockade of non-cholinergic transmitter systems should not effect processes involving memory formation and retrieval.

Cognitive Effects of Depression

The association between depression and cognitive impairment confounds assessment of TCA effects. Inclusion of impaired concentration as a criterion for major depression (American Psychiatric Association 1987) attests to the adverse impact of depression on memory. If severe, the cognitive dysfunction can reach syndromal proportions. Folstein and McHugh (1978) classify this state as a "dementia syndrome of depression" and hypothesize that catecholamine deficiencies associated with both depression and aging play a pathogenetic role. In their view, the deficits are real, measurable, and reversible. These authors eschew the term "pseudodementia," which considers the patient's state as an imitation of a true dementia.

Wells (1979) has described clinical and historical findings that distinguish pseudodementia from a state of true cognitive impairment. Wells views pseudodementia as being driven by a depressed affect that causes a subjective sense of confusion, diminished concentration, decreased motivation, and an overly pessimistic self-assessment of cognitive function. From this perspective, pseudodementia is a cognitive hypochondriasis rather than an impairment in cognitive capacity.

The term pseudodementia considers the patient's limited ability and willingness to attempt cognitive tasks as the causes of any measurable impairment in functioning. The "dementia syndrome of depression," on the other hand, speaks to a genuine inability to learn, recall, or recognize that recovers with remission of the depression. These concepts highlight the importance of distinguishing the effects of both drugs and disease on the differing components of memory functioning; specifically, inattention and poor concentration must be differentiated from an inability to learn, recall, and recognize that is not caused by deficient motivation and concentration. A systematic study of the impact of TCAs on memory must examine the effects of treatment on these differing dimensions of cognitive functioning while controlling for the contribution of affective state to performance.

Tricyclic Antidepressants, Depression, and Memory

In this section I review data that were generated from studies of the effects of depression on the subjective experience of cognitive competence, and then discuss the effects of TCAs on objective measures of the components of cognitive performance. Data from studies of geriatric depressive patients will be reviewed.

Subjective Memory and Depression

Kahn et al. (1975) have demonstrated noncongruence between self-assessment and performance in depressed subjects over age 50. Complaints of diminished memory were correlated with depression scores but not with cognitive performance; interestingly, exaggeration of complaints relative to performance was greatest in the subgroup of more depressed patients with evidence of a true concurrent cognitive deficit.

Plotkin et al. (1985), in a treatment study of depressive patients over 55 years of age, reported comparable findings on the relationship between symptoms and complaints. A decrease in memory complaints was significantly correlated with improvement in depression in both the TCA-treated individuals and the individuals who were treated with group psychotherapy.

Squire et al. (1979) developed a self-assessment test for memory and compared the effects of depression with those of bilateral electroconvulsive therapy (ECT). The kind and severity of memory complaints associated with depression differed significantly from those induced by ECT; depressed subjects gave themselves lower total memory scores than did age-matched control subjects; ECT produced lower ratings for ability to learn new material and recall recent events. Depression was associated with a particular experience of impaired ability to concentrate and sustain attention.

Components of Objective Performance

As suggested above, even the apparently straightforward cognitive function of memory involves multiple processes. These include attention, learning, retention, and the abilities to spontaneously recall and recognize. Neuropsychological tests designed to measure these functions demonstrate that Alzheimer's disease, anticholinergic drugs, and depression affect these processes differently, but that overlap does occur. For purposes of simplification, this discussion will use a model that divides memory into the categories of primary, secondary, and tertiary (Siegler and Poon 1989):

1. *Primary memory,* which involves holding onto information one has just perceived, is measured by tests that involve attention and immediate recall.
2. *Secondary memory,* which involves storage of recently learned information, is tested by serial learning, delayed recall, and delayed recognition.
3. *Tertiary, or remote, memory,* which includes items from the distant past, is least affected by the three conditions (Alzheimer's disease, TCA treatment, and depression) to be discussed.

When investigators use different terms to describe memory functions, the results will be interpreted using the model described above.

Finally a discussion of the effects of depression, anticholinergic drugs, and Alzheimer's disease on memory must consider the dimension of automatic versus effortful learning (Cohen et al. 1982; Roy-Byrne et al. 1986; Weingartner and Silberman 1984). From this perspective, depression is associated with impairment in tasks that require effortful learning and recall more than those involving automatic processing and recognition of easily learned material. Patients with Alzheimer's disease perform worse than depressive patients and control subjects on the simplest memory tests, those that involve automatic memorization without requiring organization (Weingartner and Silberman 1984). Conversely, depressive patients are specifically sensitive to tasks requiring mental effort, including organization of test material. Thus, depression has a greater impact on delayed free recall than on recognition because of the greater effort required to retrieve learned objects when a reminder is not present. Capacity to recognize uncomplicated test items involves a relatively effortless and automatic process and is most specifically affected by Alzheimer's disease.

Effects of Depression and Tricyclic Antidepressants on Cognitive Performance

Cronholm and Ottosson (1961) reported the negative impact of depression on immediate learning, but not retention, nearly 30 years ago. Subsequent studies have in a large part supported and expanded on their findings. We will review data from these studies and suggest an explanation for the selectivity of the cognitive effects of both depression and TCAs.

Henry et al. (1973), using a repeated-measures design in mixed-age adult depressive patients, found that times of increased depression were associated with decreased serial learning and free recall in unipolar subjects; however, the number of correct responses on the first trial was not affected. The authors concluded that depression interferes with serial learning as manifested by free recall (secondary memory), but not immediate (primary) memory. However, an alternative explanation is apparent. Improvement in serial learning *from the first trial* occurred after treatment with L-dopa. These results are consistent with the authors' suggestion that benefits from L-dopa result from its enervating effects; the data also suggest that depression *does* impair immediate recall (first-trial learning), and that impairment in serial learning in depressed subjects results from a carry-over of deficient initial registration (Sternberg and Jarvik 1976).

Sternberg and Jarvik (1976) carried out assessments before and after treatment in mixed-age depressive patients treated with 150 to 350 mg of amitriptyline or imipramine. Performance of the depressive patients was compared with that of age-matched control subjects. As in other studies, the principal effect of the depressed state was an interference with immediate recall. Delayed recall without the use of a reminder (more effortful secondary memory) was initially worse in depressed patients than in control subjects but was highly significantly improved after 3 weeks of TCA treatment. Delayed recall with a reminder (less effortful secondary memory) was not affected by depression. Both of these treatment studies used tertiary amine TCAs, but neither contained data that indicated a negative impact of medication treatment on measures of secondary memory.

The data from these studies provide further evidence that depression adversely affects attention and effortful cognitive tasks; furthermore, the findings indicate that the anticholinergic properties of TCAs do not disrupt secondary memory processes in mixed-age adult populations.

Prospective studies have attempted to assess the interaction between improvement in affective state and cognitive function. Glass et al. (1981), in a placebo-controlled multiple crossover design with middle-aged depressive patients, found an association between 3 weeks of treatment with 150 mg a day of imipramine and improved performance on tests involving primary memory; interestingly, no relationship was identified between affective state and performance. These data are compatible with those of Sternberg and Jarvik (1976); TCA treatment of depression leads to improvement of primary memory, presumably through increasing concentration. The Sternberg and Jarvik suggest that the lack of an association between clinical state and cognitive performance can occur because demonstrable improvement in memory precedes changes in affect as measured on depression rating scales.

Tricyclic Antidepressants and Cognitive Performance in Elderly Subjects

Two recent studies of older depressive patients provide conflicting results on the impact of TCAs on memory in this population. Georgotas et al. (1989) treated outpatient depressive patients over 55 years of age with nortriptyline, phenelzine, or placebo for 7 weeks. Patients receiving active medication demonstrated significantly greater improvement on depression ratings than did the placebo group, but were comparable on endpoint indices of cognitive functioning. Secondary memory was assessed through a paragraph-recall test and the Buschke delayed retrieval test (Buschke and Fuld 1974). No interaction was identified between clinical recovery and cognitive performance.

Hoff et al. (1990), on the other hand, did find decrements in verbal memory in an open trial of 4 weeks of nortriptyline treatment despite significant improvement in Hamilton Rating Scale for Depression scores. Interaction between clinical state and memory was not assessed. Given the differences in design, memory tests, and statistical analyses used, we are unable to reconcile these data sets.

Branconnier and coworkers (1982a, 1982b) assessed the effects of amitriptyline in geriatric depressive patients and normal elderly volunteers, respectively. The volunteer study, utilizing single doses of 50 mg of amitriptyline, demonstrated that storage (secondary learning) was not affected by the TCA but that the efficiency of retrieval by free recall was indeed profoundly impaired. It is unclear, however, whether the diminished performance resulted from sedation caused by acute treatment with amitriptyline or from an anticholinergic interference in cognitive processing. As described above (Sunderland et al. 1987), the anticholinergic activity of scopolamine interferes with storage into secondary memory; yet Branconnier et al.'s study failed to show drug-placebo differences on measures of storage or delayed recognition.

The Branconnier et al. treatment study (1982a) found elevation of a cognitive "impairment index" in elderly depressive patients treated with 150 mg of amitriptyline compared with those treated with mianserin despite similar clinical improvement; however, of the nine measures on the impairment index, only one (the Bender-Gestalt Visual Motor Test) significantly distinguished amitriptyline-treated patients. Alternative amitriptyline side effects, including impairment of psychomotor dexterity, constitute a more likely explanation for the observed decrement in performance than anticholinergic toxicity.

Data From a Discontinuation Study

We have applied a discontinuation design to examine the cognitive effects of nortriptyline in cognitively intact patients over 60 years of age who were diagnosed per DSM-III-R (American Psychiatric Association 1987) as having major depression (Meyers et al. 1990). Subjects were assessed on and off medication after 3 to 6 months of recovery from a major depressive episode to control for a contribution of depression to cognitive performance. Subjects were tapered off the concentrations (50–150 ng/ml) of nortriptyline used to treat their depression using a double-blind design. Assessments included a visual analogue version of Squire's subjective memory test (Squire et al. 1979), the Purdue Pegboard Test (Purdue Research Foundation 1948), Mattis-Kovner testing for immediate and delayed free recall (Mattis et al. 1978), and immediate and delayed recognition memory.

Our findings demonstrated that immediate free recall, but not delayed free recall or recognition, was adversely affected by nortriptyline. Medication changed the pattern of responses to Squire's 18-item self-assessment instrument (Squire et al. 1979). Subjects rated themselves significantly worse on a 9-item subset of these questions while on nortriptyline. The data suggest that therapeutic nortriptyline levels do not affect secondary-memory formation or retrieval in elderly subjects without Alzheimer's disease. We see this as being analogous to the absence of adverse cognitive effects to low doses of scopolamine in cognitively intact elderly individuals (Newhouse et al. 1988; Sunderland et al. 1987). The data can be interpreted as demonstrating an adverse effect of nortriptyline on primary memory that is associated with self-awareness of impaired performance. The absence of any effect on secondary memory, as tested by delayed free recall and recognition, suggests that secondary memory is not affected by a disturbance in the cholinergic system.

Summary

Three themes that emerged from studies published in the 1970s led to concern about the use of TCAs in elderly depressive patients:

1. Anticholinergic medications were found to impair cognitive functioning in normal volunteers.
2. Degeneration of cholinergic pathways was demonstrated as a feature of Alzheimer's disease.
3. Behavioral and cognitive disturbance occurred in a subsample of patients treated with TCAs.

The data converge in suggesting that older patients are at special risk because of putative similarities between aging-related memory impairment and cognitive disturbance caused by anticholinergic medications. The association between an increased prevalence of Alzheimer's disease and increasing age, as well as reports of a higher incidence of delirium in older patients treated with TCAs, was consistent with concern about the sensitivity of older depressive patients to the anticholinergic activity of these agents.

More recent clinical studies have enhanced our ability to use TCAs effectively while minimizing side effects. The identification of delusional depression as a disorder that can worsen when TCAs are not combined with neuroleptics, the widespread availability of testing for TCA blood levels, the identification of target levels for commonly used agents—all have helped clinicians avoid adverse behavioral effects and toxic concentrations. Furthermore, the use of secondary amine TCAs, which have less binding affinity for most neurotransmitters, especially at muscarinic sites, has increased relative to tertiary amine agents.

Components of memory function have been classified, and measures relevant to these operations have been developed. Prospective studies have assessed the contributions of age, TCA treatment, and depression to these cognitive functions. Data from these studies indicate that TCAs can be used effectively without producing clinically apparent cognitive dysfunction in the great majority of elderly depressive patients, including patients with Alzheimer's disease. Depression and acute treatment with tertiary amine TCAs *do* appear to impact on primary memory, presumably by interfering with attention and concentration. Of greater importance, long-term TCA treatment does not adversely affect the ability to store information into secondary memory or retrieve it. The absence of interference with recognition is consistent with findings from studies of low doses of scopolamine and indicates that therapeutic doses of TCAs do not produce effects similar to those of Alzheimer's disease.

Data from a discontinuation study indicate that TCAs adversely affect components of subjective memory and immediate recall, but that effects on learning and retrieval from secondary memory are minimal. Thus, patients may accurately identify decreases in memory while taking TCAs as continuation or maintenance treatment; however, these changes, like those after ECT, are not demonstrable on measurements of learning and secondary memory.

Early concerns that elderly patients would develop confusional syndromes during treatment with TCAs were exaggerated. The anticholinergic activity of these agents, especially the secondary amines, when administered at therapeutic serum levels is not sufficient to disrupt long-term memory in a meaningful way. Nevertheless, elderly subjects do experience subjective impairment when given TCAs, and this may be related to an actual deficit in short-term recall. Further studies are required to clarify the impact of standard clinical concentrations of TCAs on the different components of memory and on the relationship between these effects and the anticholinergic activity of these agents.

References

American Psychiatric Association: Diagnostic and Statistical Manual of Mental Disorders, 3rd Edition, Revised. Washington, DC, American Psychiatric Association, 1987

American Psychiatric Association Task Force on the Use of Laboratory Tests in Psychiatry: Tricyclic antidepressants—blood level measurements and clinical outcome: an APA Task Force report. Am J Psychiatry 142:149–162, 1985

Åsberg M, Cronholm B, Sjoquist F, et al: Relationship between plasma level and therapeutic effect of nortriptyline. Br Med J 3:331–334, 1971

Bartus RT, Dean RL III, Beer B, et al: The cholinergic hypothesis of geriatric memory dysfunction. Science 217:408–417, 1982

Blessed G, Tomlinson BE, Roth M: The association between quantitative measures of dementia and of senile changes in the grey matter of elderly subjects. Br J Psychiatry 114:797-811, 1968

Branconnier RJ, Cole JO, Ghazvinian S, et al: Treating the depressed elderly patient: the comparative behavioral pharmacology of mianserin and amitriptyline, in Typical and Atypical Antidepressants: Clinical Practice. Edited by Costa E, Racagni G. New York, Raven, 1982a

Branconnier RJ, DeVitt DR, Cole JO, et al: Amitriptyline selectively disrupts verbal recall from secondary memory of the normal aged. Neurobiol Aging 3:55–59, 1982b

Buschke H, Fuld P: Evaluating storage, retention, and retrieval in disordered memory and learning. Neurology 24:1019–1025, 1974

Cohen, RM, Weingartner H, Smallberg SA, et al: Effort and cognition in depression. Arch Gen Psychiatry 39:593–597, 1982

Cronholm B, Ottosson JO: Memory functions in endogenous depression. Archives of General Depression 5:101–107, 1961

Davies P: Loss of choline acetyltransferase activity in normal aging and in senile dementia. Adv Exper Med Biol 113:251–256 1978

Davies P, Maloney AJF: Selective loss of central cholinergic neurons in Alzheimer's disease. Lancet 2:1403, 1976

Davies RK, Tucker GJ, Harrow M, et al: Confusional episodes and antidepressant medication. Am J Psychiatry 128:95–99[127–131], 1971

Drachman DA: Memory and cognitive function in man: does the cholinergic system have a specific role? Neurology 27:783–790, 1977

Drachman DA, Leavitt J: Human memory and the cholinergic system: a relationship to aging? Arch Neurol 30:113–121, 1974

Folstein MF, McHugh PR: Dementia syndrome of depression, in Alzheimer's Disease: Senile Dementia and Related Disorders. Edited by Katzman R, Terry RD, Bick KL. New York, Raven, 1978, pp 87–96

Folstein MF, Folstein SE, McHugh PR: "Mini-Mental State": a practical method for grading the cognitive state of patients for the clinician. J Psychiatr Res 12:189–198, 1975

Georgotas A, McCue RE, Reisberg B, et al: The effects of mood changes and antidepressants on the cognitive capacity of elderly depressed patients. International Psychogeriatrics 1:135–143, 1986

Glass RM, Uhlenhuth EH, Hartel FW, et al: Cognitive dysfunction and imipramine in outpatient depressives. Arch Gen Psychiatry 38:1048–1051, 1981

Henry GM, Weingartner H, Murphy D: Influence of affective states and psychoactive drugs on verbal learning and memory. Am J Psychiatry 130:966–971, 1973

Hoff AL, Shukla S, Helms P, et al: The effects of nortriptyline on cognition in elderly depressed patients (letter). J Clin Psychopharmacol 10:231–232, 1990

Jenike MA: Handbook of Geriatric Psychiatry. Littleton, MA, PSG Publishing, 1985

Kahn RL, Zarit SH, Hilbert NM, et al: Memory complaint and impairment in the aged: the effect of depression and altered brain function. Arch Gen Psychiatry 32:1569–1573, 1975

Ketchum JS, Sidell FR, Crowell EB Jr, et al: Atropine, scopolamine and ditran: comparative pharmacology and antagonists in man. Psychopharmacology (Berlin) 28:121–145, 1973

Livingston RL, Zucker DK, Isenberg K, et al: Tricyclic antidepressants and delirium. J Clin Psychiatry 44(5):173–176, 1983

Mattis S, Kovner R, Goldmeier E: Different patterns of mnemonic deficits in two organic syndromes. Brain Lang 6:179–191, 1978

Meador-Woodruff JH, Akil M, Wisner-Carlson R, et al: Behavioral and cognitive toxicity related to elevated plasma tricyclic antidepressant levels. J Clin Psychopharmacol 8:28–32, 1988

Meyers BS, Mei-Tal V: Psychiatric reactions during tricyclic treatment of the elderly reconsidered. J Clin Psychopharmacol 3:2–6, 1983

Meyers BS, Mei-Tal V: Empirical study on an inpatient psychogeriatric unit: biological treatment in patients with depressive illness. Int J Psychiatry Med 15:111–124, 1985–1986

Meyers BS, Mattis S, Gabriele M, et al: Nortriptyline and memory in elderly depressives: comparison of objective and subjective effects. Poster presented at the annual meeting of the American College of Neuropharmacology, San Juan, Puerto Rico, December 1990

Nelson JC, Bowers MB Jr, Sweeney DR: Exacerbation of psychosis by tricyclic antidepressants in delusional depression. Am J Psychiatry 136:574–576, 1979

Nelson JC, Jatlow P, Mazure C: Desipramine plasma levels and response in elderly melancholic patients. J Clin Psychopharmacol 5:217–220, 1985

Newhouse PA, Sunderland T, Tariot PN, et al: The effects of acute scopolamine in geriatric depression. Arch Gen Psychiatry 45:906–912, 1988

Nies A, Robinson DS, Friedman MJ, et al: Relationship between age and tricyclic antidepressant plasma levels. Am J Psychiatry 134:790–793, 1977

Perry EK, Perry RH, Blessed G, et al: Necropsy evidence of central cholinergic deficits in senile dementia. Lancet 1:189, 1977

Plotkin DA, Mintz J, Jarvik LF: Subjective memory complaints in geriatric depression. Am J Psychiatry 142:1103–1105, 1985

Preskorn SH, Simpson S: Tricyclic antidepressant induced delirium and plasma drug concentrations. Am J Psychiatry 139:822–823, 1982

Purdue Research Foundation: Examiner's Manual for the Purdue Pegboard. Chicago, IL, Science Research Associates, 1948

Reifler BV, Teri L, Raskind M: Double-blind trial of imipramine in Alzheimer's disease patients with and without depression. Am J Psychiatry 146:45–49, 1989

Reynolds CF III, Perel JM, Kupfer DJ, et al: Open-trial response to antidepressant treatment in elderly patients with mixed depression and cognitive impairment. Psychiatry Res 21:111–122, 1987

Richelson E: Pharmacology of antidepressants in use in the United States. J Clin Psychiatry 43(11, sec 2):4–11, 1982

Roy-Byrne PP, Weingartner H, Bierer LM, et al: Effortful and automatic cognitive processes in depression. Arch Gen Psychiatry 43:265–267, 1986

Safer DJ, Allen RP: The central effects of scopolamine in man. Biol Psychiatry 3:347–355, 1971

Siegler IC, Poon LW: The psychology of aging, in Geriatric Psychiatry. Edited by Busse EW, Blazer DG. Washington, DC, American Psychiatric Press, 1989, pp 163–201

Smith CM, Swash M: Possible biochemical basis of memory disorder in Alzheimer disease. Ann Neurol 3:471–473, 1978

Snyder SH, Yamamura HI: Antidepressants and the muscarinic acetylcholine receptor. Arch Gen Psychiatry 34:236–239, 1977

Squire LR, Wetzel CD, Slater PC: Memory complaint after electroconvulsive therapy: assessment with a new self-rating instrument. Biol Psychiatry 14:791–801, 1979

Sternberg DE, Jarvik ME: Memory functions in depression: improvement with antidepressant medication. Arch Gen Psychiatry 33:219–224, 1976

Sunderland T, Tariot PN, Cohen RM, et al: Anticholinergic sensitivity in patients with dementia of the Alzheimer type and age-matched controls. Arch Gen Psychiatry 44:418–426, 1987

Szabadi E, Gaszner P, Bradshaw CM: The peripheral anticholinergic activity of tricyclic antidepressants: comparison of amitriptyline and desipramine in human volunteers. Br J Psychiatry 137:433–439, 1980

Weingartner H, Silberman E: Cognitive changes in depression, in Neurobiology of Mood Disorders. Edited by Post RM, Ballenger JC. Baltimore, MD, Williams & Wilkins, 1984, pp 121–135

Wells CE: Pseudodementia. Am J Psychiatry 136:895–900, 1979

Whitehouse PJ, Price DL, Clark AW, et al: Alzheimer disease: evidence for selective loss of cholinergic neurons in the nucleus basalis. Ann Neurol 10:122–126, 1980

Chapter 2

Cardiac Risks of Antidepressants in the Elderly

Marcella Pascualy, M.D.
M. Michele Murburg, M.D.
Richard C. Veith, M.D.

Shortly after the tricyclic antidepressants (TCAs) achieved widespread clinical use, it became apparent that they were potentially lethal following overdose and that the morbidity of these agents in the overdose setting was largely attributable to cardiovascular toxicity. This knowledge created a dilemma for clinicians caring for elderly patients or for those patients with significant cardiac disease, because it was assumed that such individuals were at increased risk to develop cardiovascular adverse effects during routine clinical treatment with these agents. Fortunately, clinical research conducted over the past 15 years has demonstrated that the serious cardiovascular complications associated with TCA poisoning do not necessarily apply to patients, even those with compromised cardiovascular functioning, who are treated with the usual doses employed in the therapeutic setting. Although important questions remain unanswered, recent clinical research has clarified the risks of treating the elderly. The purpose of this chapter is to provide a review of the cardiovascular properties of commonly employed antidepressant agents and to offer guidelines for the treatment of individuals who, because of advanced age, might be considered at increased risk for cardiovascular complications during antidepressant treatment.

This work was supported by the Medical Research Service of the Department of Veterans Affairs.

Cardiovascular Effects of Antidepressant Overdose: Historical Perspective

Approximately 5,000 to 10,000 people in the United States poison themselves with a TCA annually (Moriarty 1981). Cardiotoxicity is a major complication of TCA overdose and is often the cause of death in this setting. The most common cardiovascular manifestations of TCA overdose are tachycardia and hypotension (Goldberg et al. 1985; Langou et al. 1980). Of greater concern in the management of overdose patients, however, is the development of conduction and repolarization disturbances that often accompany TCA poisoning. Conduction disturbances may manifest themselves electrocardiographically as prolongation of the PR interval, QRS interval, or QT_c interval (QT interval corrected for heart rate). In the most severe situation, atrioventricular block, ventricular arrhythmias, and ultimately asystole cardiovascular collapse and death, may occur. Complications are most prevalent in patients who achieve plasma levels in excess of 1,000 pg/ml (Spiker et al. 1975). Because plasma level measurements are not routinely available in the acute overdose setting, and because some studies have failed to find them of predictive value (Boehnert and Lovejoy 1985), plasma level monitoring has not proven to be useful in the management of most overdose patients. One study indicated that the presence of QRS duration greater than 100 milliseconds is predictive of ventricular arrhythmias and seizures following overdose (Boehnert and Lovejoy 1985). Because the QRS duration can be easily obtained from the electrocardiogram (ECG), this measure has been advocated for identifying those individuals most likely to develop serious complications following TCA poisoning. However, this finding has been disputed (Foulke and Albertson 1987).

Characteristically, the serious cardiovascular complications of TCA overdose are dose-related and are clinically evident within the first 24 hours after poisoning occurs. Goldberg et al. (1985) reported that in a series of 75 overdose cases, none of their patients who had regained consciousness and had a normal electrocardiogram for 24 hours went on to develop any significant arrhythmia. Thus, elaborate cardiovascular monitoring may be of limited value beyond this point.

In view of the seriousness of the cardiovascular consequences of TCA overdose and in the absence of evidence to the contrary, it is not surprising that in the 1960s and 1970s the antidepressants developed a reputation for being potentially hazardous for depressed patients who were elderly or had heart disease. This concern was amplified by reports in the early 1970s of unexplained sudden death in medically ill patients who were receiving customary clinical doses of these agents. Undoubtedly, one unfortunate consequence of the fears generated by such reports was a reluctance by clinicians to offer TCA treatment to elderly or medically ill patients. The 1977 report by Bigger et al. (1977) that typical, therapeutic doses of imipramine were effective in *reducing* ventricular arrhythmias forced a reappraisal of the cardiovascular risks of therapeutic doses of the TCAs. Subsequent clinical research has clarified the potential cardiovascular risks of TCA treatment of the elderly patient and is the focus of this review.

Pharmacological Properties of the Tricyclic Antidepressants: Potential Effects on Cardiovascular Regulation

As a group, the TCAs exhibit pharmacological properties that would be expected to influence cardiovascular function through actions at several physiological sites. Possible mechanisms include actions in brain regions important in regulating cardiovascular homeostasis; influences on sympathetic and parasympathetic neural regulation of the heart; direct receptor effects in cardiac tissue and on peripheral blood vessels as well as influences on local neurotransmitter availability at these receptor sites; alterations of circulating plasma norepinephrine concentrations with resulting hormonal effects on end-organ adrenergic receptors; and direct actions at the cellular level in the myocardium.

Prevailing theories suggest that the TCAs exert their therapeutic effects through effects on noradrenergic, serotonergic, and/or cholinergic neurotransmitter systems in the brain. It is also likely that central nervous system (CNS) actions are responsible, in part, for the cardiovascular effects of these agents. For example, cell groups in the rostral ventrolateral medulla integrate descending cortical and hypothalamic input, autonomic efferent activity, and afferent feedback from peripheral baroreceptors, and closely regulate central input to the cardiovascular system (Reis et al. 1988). The TCAs likely act on the receptors for norepinephrine, serotonin, and acetylcholine that have been identified in these brain regions and on the neuronal pathways utilizing these neurotransmitters that form an important part of the CNS network regulating cardiovascular and hemodynamic functioning (Reis et al. 1988; Sawchenko et al. 1987).

One mechanism by which the CNS effects of the TCAs would be transmitted to the heart is via the sympathetic and parasympathetic systems. Activation of the sympathetic pathways innervating the heart increases the rate and force of cardiac contraction through the local release of norepinephrine. Norepinephrine released from postganglionic sympathetic nerves also stimulates postsynaptic $alpha_1$ and $alpha_2$ adrenergic receptors on peripheral arteries, causing vasoconstriction and increased blood pressure. Parasympathetic input to the heart, transmitted through the vagus nerve, slows heart rate through increased impulse flow and increases heart rate by withdrawal of vagal impulse traffic. Afferent input to the medullary cardiovascular centers is transmitted from the baroreceptors via the glossopharyngeal and vagus nerves, thereby completing the reflex loop of CNS blood pressure regulation.

Neuroendocrine factors, including alterations in sympathetic and parasympathetic input, interact with intrinsic cardiac mechanisms in a complex array of counter-regulatory systems to control cardiac rate, rhythm, output, and blood pressure. The sinoatrial node, normally the pacemaker for the heart, sends impulses down the atrial internodal tracts, depolarizing the atria. Depolarization of the atria, associated with the P wave of the ECG, is followed by contraction of the atria as the impulse travels through the atrioventricular node. From the atrioventricular node, the impulse enters the bundle of His, which divides into the right and left bundle branches. These, in turn, divide progressively into a conduction network of Purkinje fibers, stimulation of which causes contraction of the ventricular muscle. Depolarization of the ventricle is seen on the ECG as the QRS complex. Repolarization of the ventricles is reflected in the QT interval, which represents the time from the beginning of ventricular depolarization through completion of ventricular repolarization.

Because, to varying degrees, the TCAs bind to noradrenergic and cholinergic receptors in the periphery as well as in the brain, it is also likely that they influence cardiovascular function through direct binding effects on adrenergic and cholinergic receptors on sympathetic nerves, the adrenal medulla, and peripheral blood vessels, and in cardiac tissue. In addition, it has been demonstrated that prolonged TCA treatment increases circulating plasma norepinephrine concentrations (Veith et al. 1983), and, by the norepinephrine acting as a circulating hormone rather than as a neurotransmitter, this effect might be expected to increase cardiovascular responses by activation of peripheral adrenergic receptors. It is presently unclear whether the TCA-induced rise in plasma norepinephrine concentration following prolonged TCA treatment represents an increase in sympathetic activity or is the result of reuptake blockade of norepinephrine at peripheral noradrenergic neurons, which also would be expected to increase plasma norepinephrine concentrations. Studies employing tritiated norepinephrine isotope dilution techniques to measure plasma norepinephrine kinetics would be required to resolve this question, and such studies are underway presently in our laboratories. However, it is also important to note that, in the absence of unusually elevated pretreatment plasma norepinephrine concentrations, the modest elevation in plasma norepinephrine associated with TCA administration would not be likely to have any meaningful physiological effect on cardiovascular function, because it has previously been shown, using infusions of exogenous norepinephrine, that an approximately eightfold increase in circulating norepinephrine concentrations is required to produce changes in blood pressure or heart rate (Silverberg et al. 1978).

The TCAs tend to be highly concentrated in cardiac tissue and have been shown to produce a dose-dependent shortening of Purkinje fiber action-potential duration and a reduction in Purkinje fiber and ventricular muscle action-potential upstroke velocity (Muir et al. 1982; Soroko and Maxwell 1983; Weld and Bigger 1980). These effects are evident at concentrations considered therapeutic in humans. At clinically toxic levels in humans, the TCAs have been shown to suppress spontaneous firing of canine Purkinje fibers, which can ultimately cause complete blockade of transmembrane potentials in papillary muscle (Muir et al. 1982; Soroko and Maxwell 1983; Weld and Bigger 1980). This direct electrical suppression of the ventricular tissue may account for the conduction defects and arrhythmias seen during TCA toxicity in humans.

Cardiovascular Effects of Customary Doses of the Tricyclic Antidepressants

Effects on the Electrocardiogram and Intraventricular Conduction

The TCAs tend to slow intracardiac conduction and produce a variety of electrocardiographic changes. Although there have been few studies of exclusively elderly patients that have examined the relationship between therapeutically effective doses of the TCA and their effects on the ECG, it can generally be expected that patients receiving customary outpatient doses of a TCA will exhibit an increase in heart rate of 5–15 beats/minute. In the absence of orthostatic hypotension, which would also be expected to increase heart rate via baroreceptor mechanisms, this increase in heart rate is presumably due primarily to the anticholinergic properties of the TCA. CNS anticholinergic effects would be expected to diminish vagally mediated restraint on sinus node firing rate, resulting in an increase in heart rate. An increase in heart rate exceeding 100 beats/minute should be considered unusual and should warrant an exploration for an alternative explanation. TCA-induced increases in heart rate are generally well tolerated, if the patient is informed that this effect might accompany treatment.

In young, healthy individuals receiving customary doses of the TCAs, prolongation of the PR interval, the QRS interval, and the QT_C interval is frequently observed (Glassman and Bigger 1981; Luchins 1983; Veith et al. 1982a). Clinical studies reveal only a weak correlation between TCA-induced ECG changes and plasma TCA concentrations (Glassman and Bigger 1981; Veith et al. 1982a). Such alterations in the ECG are generally not clinically important in healthy patients, and the prolongation of these parameters does not usually exceed the upper limits of normal values.

The significance of these changes, however, is that they reflect the potential of these agents to delay intracardiac conduction. Animal and human studies indicate that the TCAs delay intraventricular conduction by prolonging transit of electrical impulses through the distal Purkinje specialized conducting system of the ventricles (Burrows et al. 1977; Soroko and Maxwell 1983; Weld and Bigger 1980). This effect is reversible, appears to be dose-related, and is a property shared by all of the first-generation TCAs (i.e., amitriptyline, imipramine, nortriptyline, protriptyline, doxepin, and desipramine). Throughout the 1960s and 1970s, clinical lore suggested that doxepin produced fewer effects on cardiovascular functioning than the other first-generation TCAs. However, careful review of the animal and clinical literature indicates that this impression was unwarranted (Luchins 1983).

The major concern, of course, is that this effect of the TCAs may exacerbate preexisting conduction disturbances in elderly patients with known or occult heart disease. Indeed, several case reports have documented the ability of these agents to produce a high degree of heart block in such individuals (Kantor et al. 1975; Roose et al. 1987b; Smith and Rusbatch 1967; Stoudemire and Atkinson 1988). It would be clinically useful to identify those individuals who might be susceptible to this potentially life-threatening adverse response and to determine the relationship between preexisting conduction disturbances and TCA-induced cardiovascular complications. These questions were recently addressed in a study by Roose et al. (1987b), who reported on 42 patients with conduction abnormalities who were treated with imipramine and/or nortriptyline. Of the 11 patients with pretreatment first-degree heart block (PR interval duration greater than 100 milliseconds), none developed further complications within a range of plasma concentrations of imipramine plus desipramine of 315 ± 102 ng/ml or nortriptyline of 98 ± 17 ng/ml. In contrast, of the 30 patients with pretreatment bundle branch block, 2 developed 2:1 atrioventricular block, 2 developed greater than a 25% increase in QRS duration, 2 had a sinus arrest, and 1 experienced a myocardial infarction. The small sample size in this study limits the interpretation of these findings, but this work suggests that the presence of a first-degree heart block is not a serious concern for patients receiving a TCA(s). Although it is possible that some of the complications observed in the patients with pretreatment bundle branch block were not causally related to TCA administration (i.e., there was no untreated control group to determine the naturalistic rate of the development of these problems attributable to the presence of heart disease alone), the Roose et al. (1987b) data suggest that the first-generation TCAs should be avoided in patients with significant conduction abnormalities or that such patients should be treated in a setting where they can be closely monitored. It should be noted in this context that the monoamine oxidase (MAO) inhibitors do not delay intraventricular conduction and, thus, might prove to be a useful alternative treatment for such individuals. In addition, both fluoxetine and bupropion appear to be less likely than the first-generation TCAs to affect conduction (see below).

Effects on Cardiac Rhythm

Serious cardiac arrhythmias can occur following TCA poisoning. In addition, case reports suggest that some individuals are susceptible to arrhythmias during routine clinical treatment with the TCAs. However, it is now apparent that the usual effect of typical outpatient doses of the

TCAs in the majority of patients is an antiarrhythmic effect. This was first demonstrated in 1977 by Bigger et al. (1977), who observed a reduction in premature ventricular complexes in two elderly cardiac patients treated with imipramine. In 1978, Wilkerson (1978) demonstrated that the TCAs effectively prevented experimentally induced cardiac arrhythmias in doses comparable to and slightly above those used clinically. It has subsequently been confirmed in human and animal studies that the suppressant effect of the TCAs on ventricular automaticity is equal to or greater than that associated with quinidine and procainamide, class 1 antiarrhythmic drugs (Soroko and Maxwell 1983; Weld and Bigger 1980). A direct antiarrhythmic effect has been demonstrated in humans for imipramine, nortriptyline, doxepin, and maprotiline (Bigger et al. 1977; Connolly et al. 1984; Giardina and Bigger 1982; Giardina et al. 1986, 1987; Raeder et al. 1979; Veith et al. 1982b). In fact, a careful examination of the ECG and the electrophysiological data from available human and animal studies suggests that the first-generation TCAs should all share this property. In summary, it is now generally accepted that although individual patients will occasionally develop rhythm disturbances with the use of the first-generation TCAs, it should generally be expected that an antiarrhythmic effect will be the usual response in most patients receiving customary clinical doses of these agents.

Effects on Myocardial Performance

Prior to the 1980s, conventional clinical wisdom suggested that the TCAs were capable of exacerbating hemodynamic and myocardial performance in individuals with impaired ventricular function. In part, this impression was an additional legacy of the cardiotoxicity associated with TCA poisoning. It had also been reported that the TCAs had a direct myocardial depressant effect in animal studies, but this occurs in doses and plasma level ranges that are clearly toxic for humans. In addition, several investigators suggested that the TCAs reduced myocardial contractility, because it had been observed that systolic time intervals (simultaneous recording of the ECG, phonocardiogram, and the carotid pulse wave) were prolonged in patients receiving therapeutic doses of the TCAs. However, systolic time intervals can be influenced by such factors as bundle branch block or other intraventricular conduction delay. Thus, it is likely that the changes in systolic time intervals, interpreted as evidence of a TCA-induced negative inotropic effect, were instead a reflection of the prolongation of intraventricular conduction that frequently accompanies treatment with these agents.

In 1982, Veith et al. (1982b) employed radionuclide techniques to measure the left ventricular ejection fraction, a sensitive index of myocardial performance, in depressed patients with cardiac disease who were subsequently treated with therapeutically effective doses of imipramine or doxepin. These investigators found no adverse effect of the TCAs on the myocardial performance at rest or during maximal bicycle exercise. Although the statistical power of the double-blind, placebo-controlled study was sufficient to detect a clinically meaningful change in left ventricular performance, it was acknowledged that the sample size was small, that the doses employed were relatively modest, and that few of the patients treated with the active agents had severe impairment of left ventricular function. Glassman and associates subsequently confirmed these findings of Veith et al. in a series of studies in patients with more severe cardiac disease who were treated with higher doses of imipramine or nortriptyline and at correspondingly greater plasma concentrations (Glassman et al. 1983; Roose et al. 1986, 1987a). It is now generally accepted that in customary clinical doses, the first-generation TCAs do not significantly interfere with left ventricular pump function.

Although these studies found no adverse effect of TCA administration on myocardial performance in patients with cardiac disease, it should not be concluded that treatment of such patients is without hazards. In addition to the concerns related to conduction delay noted above, both the study by Veith et al. (1982b) and those by Glassman and associates (Glassman et al. 1983; Roose et al. 1987a) suggest that cardiac patients may be particularly prone to postural hypotension from TCA treatment (see below).

Effects on Blood Pressure

Perhaps the most frequent serious hemodynamic complication of TCA therapy is postural hypotension. Approximately 20% of patients will experience orthostatic hypotension, with an even greater frequency and increased severity occurring in patients with cardiac disease and in those with preexisting orthostasis (Glassman and Bigger 1981; Glassman et al. 1979; Roose et al. 1981, 1987a, 1987b). The mechanism by which the TCAs produce orthostasis is not established, but antagonism of alpha-adrenergic receptors on the peripheral vasculature is a popular explanation.

The relative importance of such apparent risk factors as preexisting cardiac disease, antidepressant dose, plasma concentration, and specific drug selection in determining the emergence of clinically significant orthostatic hypotension with the administration of TCAs is not completely clear. Glassman et al. (1979) reported that, in their experience, imipramine-induced orthostatic hypotension occurs early in treatment and is not worsened by increasing doses or higher blood levels. It is important to note, however, that this orthostatic hypotension occurred in the context of rapid dosing increments to high dose levels. Nelson et al. (1985) reported that significant orthostatic hypotension can occur at a relatively low plasma TCA concentration in elderly patients.

We, too, have had this experience, but in contrast to Glassman et al. (1979), we have also observed many patients in whom the emergence of orthostasis appeared to be dose-related and seemed to resolve with dose reduction.

Glassman et al. (1983) have proposed that the presence of depression in cardiac patients imparts an increased risk for orthostasis, because the depressed cardiac patients who were studied (Glassman et al. 1983) had greater blood pressure difficulties than did a group of nondepressed cardiac patients (Giardina and Bigger 1982). However, the plasma TCA levels averaged 388 ± 190 ng/ml in the depressed cardiac patients and only 172 ± 59 ng/ml in the nondepressed patients, raising the possibility that the difference in plasma levels, not the presence of depression, was responsible for the more severe orthostasis of the former group. This interpretation is further strengthened by the fact that the orthostatic responses of the depressed patients in the study by Veith et al. (1982b) were quite similar to those of the nondepressed cardiac patients of the Giardina and Bigger (1982) study, and these responses were associated with similar plasma TCA concentrations in the two studies.

Roose et al. (1981) reported that nortriptyline was significantly less likely than imipramine to produce orthostatic hypotension. This was also reported by Thayssen et al. (1981) in a group of elderly (age 62–78 years) patients. In both studies, plasma nortriptyline concentrations were lower than the plasma concentrations for imipramine, raising the likelihood that the lower plasma concentrations required for therapeutic effects, rather than inherent pharmacological differences, account for the apparent advantage of using nortriptyline in high-risk patients. Finally, Roose et al. (1987b) have also reported an increased risk for orthostatic hypotension in patients with preexisting cardiac conduction abnormalities.

Cardiovascular Effects of the Second-Generation Antidepressants

Five antidepressants have been released in the United States market over the past 10 years that have structures or pharmacological profiles that distinguish them from the first-generation antidepressants. Several of these agents also appear to differ from the early antidepressants in their cardiovascular profiles, raising the potential that these agents might be preferred when treating elderly patients.

Maprotiline

Although this agent is distinct as the one tetracyclic antidepressant currently available, it is similar to imipramine, desipramine, and nortriptyline in that it is a potent inhibitor of norepinephrine neuronal uptake. Its affinity for human caudate acetylcholine receptors is approximately one-third that of desipramine (Richelson 1984). Maprotiline is also similar to the first-generation agents in terms of its cardiovascular profile.

Animal and clinical studies indicate that maprotiline increases heart rate, lengthens the PR, QRS, and QT_c intervals, and produces orthostatic hypotension (Ahles et al. 1984; Brorson and Wennerblom 1982; Edwards and Goldie 1983; Lindbom et al. 1982; Raeder et al. 1979). As is true for the first-generation TCAs, the quinidine-like tendency of maprotiline to delay cardiac conduction is also associated with the potential to suppress ventricular arrhythmias in humans (Ahles et al. 1984; Raeder et al. 1979). In summary, maprotiline has a cardiovascular profile quite similar to those of the first-generation TCAs.

Trazodone

Trazodone is a triazolopyridine derivative that selectively inhibits neuronal uptake of serotonin (Clements-Jewry et al. 1980; Riblet et al. 1979) and has both serotonin agonist and antagonist properties (Maj et al. 1979). In addition, trazodone binds strongly to cortical alpha$_1$ receptors, an effect correlated clinically with a tendency to cause sedation and hypotension (Clements-Jewry et al. 1980). Unlike the first-generation antidepressants, trazodone has only weak antihistaminic and anticholinergic effects (Clements-Jewry et al. 1980).

The cardiovascular effects of trazodone have been well studied in animals but somewhat less extensively so in humans. The lethal dose of trazodone is approximately three times higher than that of imipramine in rats (Lisciani et al. 1978). In doses comparable to those used clinically in humans, trazodone causes hypotension and delays atrial conduction in animals (Gomoll et al. 1979; Lisciani et al. 1978). In contrast to the first-generation TCAs, trazodone administered intravenously does not delay intraventricular cardiac conduction or produce significant electrocardiographic changes in dogs (Byrne and Gomoll 1982). In overdose situations, trazodone has been reported not to have significant cardiovascular toxicity (Henry et al. 1984).

In studies involving normal human subjects, trazodone, 10 mg po given as a single dose, significantly decreased heart rate and diastolic blood pressure and had no effect on stroke volume or cardiac output (Hames et al. 1982). In doses of 150–400 mg in depressed patients, trazodone did not alter PR, QRS, or QT intervals (Hayes et al. 1983; Robinson et al. 1984). In a group of depressed elderly patients (Hayes et al. 1983), trazodone at a mean dose of 305 mg daily did not alter heart rate or intracardiac conduction. Five of 19 patients developed transient ST-segment depression, and two developed persistent ST-segment suppression, but none were symptomatic.

In recent years, disturbances of cardiac rhythm and conduction have been reported in association with trazodone use. Reports of increased ventricular ectopy (Aronson and Hafez 1986; Himmelhoch 1981; Himmelhoch et al. 1984; Janowsky et al. 1983), exacerbation of ventricular tachycardia (Vlay and Friedling 1983), atrial fibrillation (White and Wong 1985), complete heart block (Rausch et al. 1984), first-degree heart block, and junctional bradycardia (Irwin and Spar 1983) have been described that were thought to be reversibly related to trazodone use. However, one placebo-controlled, double-blind study found no difference between trazodone and placebo in increasing premature ventricular contractions in a group of depressed patients with a variety of cardiovascular disorders (Lippmann 1985).

In summary, trazodone clearly has fewer anticholinergic effects than the first-generation TCAs. It tends to slow heart rate and can produce orthostatic hypotension. In both animals and humans, trazodone has been found to prolong ventricular repolarization. Some patients with preexisting ventricular arrhythmias may experience an exacerbation of these problems, and other patients with prolonged PR intervals at baseline have been reported to show further prolongation with trazodone administration. However, although these case reports suggest that patients with cardiac disease should be treated cautiously with trazodone, an increase in arrhythmias or worsening of conduction disturbances has not yet been demonstrated in controlled studies. Animal studies and clinical reports suggest a more benign cardiovascular effect of trazodone following overdose.

Amoxapine

Amoxapine is a member of the dibenzoxazepine subclass of TCAs, with a neuropharmacological and clinical profile sufficiently distinct from those of the first-generation TCAs to warrant discussion. Both amoxapine and its 7-hydroxyamine metabolite have been shown in radioreceptor assays to have plasma neuroleptic activities comparable to those of typical neuroleptics. Not surprisingly, side effects consistent with dopamine blockade, including hyperprolactinemia, galactorrhea, dystonia, akathisia, tardive dyskinesia, and neuroleptic malignant syndrome have been reported with the use of amoxapine. (Frankly, we are aware of no sufficiently compelling differential benefit of the use of this agent that justifies exposing depressed patients to the risk of tardive dyskinesia.)

Amoxapine and its active metabolites block neuronal reuptake of norepinephrine and, to a lesser extent, serotonin (Coupet et al. 1979; Greenblatt et al. 1978). On the basis of preclinical studies, amoxapine was reported to have relatively weak CNS, but significant peripheral, anticholinergic properties (Greenblatt et al. 1978).

Despite early marketing claims to the contrary, the cardiovascular profile of amoxapine appears to be similar to those of the other TCAs. Amoxapine, like imipramine and amitriptyline, causes an increase in heart rate consistent with its adrenergic and anticholinergic actions, and it causes orthostatic hypotension in approximately 40% of patients (Robinson et al. 1984). The electrocardiographic effects noted with amoxapine include tachycardia and nonspecific T-wave changes similar to those seen with the other TCAs. Although one study reported a reduction in QRS interval (Robinson et al. 1984), altered repolarization, first-degree heart block, and bundle branch block have been reported (Charalampous 1972; Hertzman and Goins 1984; Zavodnick 1981), suggesting similarities between amoxapine and the other TCAs. One large study reported a decrease in QT interval with amoxapine (Robinson et al. 1984), but the findings from this study were not corrected for increased heart rate, which shortens the QT interval.

Amoxapine overdose frequently causes acute renal failure (often apparently related to rhabdomyolysis and myoglobinurea) and seizures (Kulig et al. 1982; Pumariega et al. 1982). Cardiovascular complications reported in the setting of oliguric renal failure caused by amoxapine overdose include sinus tachycardia, congestive heart failure, and hypertension (Kulig et al. 1982; Pumariega et al. 1982). In 5 patients, amoxapine overdose was associated with no electrocardiographic or cardiovascular abnormalities (Kulig et al. 1982), and this was the foundation for the claims of fewer cardiovascular effects of amoxapine compared with the other TCAs. In a series of 33 patients (Litovitz and Troutman 1983), supraventricular tachycardia was found in 13 patients and respiratory depression and hypotension in 7 patients following amoxapine overdose.

In summary, amoxapine shares with other TCAs a propensity to cause anticholinergic side effects, tachycardia, postural hypotension, and nonspecific T-wave changes on the ECG. Amoxapine, like the other TCAs, probably prolongs intraventricular conduction, but definitive descriptions comparing the effects of amoxapine to other TCAs with regard to cardiac conduction or rhythm have not been published. The effects of toxic or therapeutic doses of amoxapine on left ventricular performance in patients with cardiac disease are unknown. Current evidence does suggest, however, that amoxapine is less directly cardiotoxic than the other TCAs following overdose.

Bupropion

Bupropion is an aminoketone derivative that is chemically distinct from the TCAs, the MAO inhibitors, and other "second-generation" antidepressants. The mechanisms by which bupropion exerts its antidepressant effects are not clear. In therapeutic concentrations, it has no significant effects on norepinephrine or serotonin reuptake and release, it does not affect MAO A or MAO B, it is not a sympathomimetic, and it is not anticholinergic (Ferns et al. 1978; Leighton and Maxwell 1978; Soroko and Maxwell 1983). Although it has mild stimulant properties (Soroko and Maxwell 1983), it does not significantly stimulate the release of norepinephrine, dopamine, or serotonin from synaptosomal preparations (Ferns et al. 1978).

From these features of the pharmacology of bupropion, one might predict relatively fewer cardiovascular effects compared with the first-generation TCAs. Indeed, animal studies indicate that bupropion is approximately 10-fold weaker than the TCAs as a cardiac depressant (Soroko and Maxwell 1983). Bolus injections of bupropion, 5–10 mg/kg, caused transient decreases in mean arterial pressure and increases in heart rate without significant electrocardiographic changes in dogs (Soroko and Maxwell 1983). Oral doses of bupropion as high as 25 mg/kg had no effect on blood pressure but caused a sustained 20% increase in heart rate (Soroko and Maxwell 1983).

In normal human subjects, bupropion in single oral doses from 5 to 800 mg caused either no effect or a modest increase in heart rate and no effect on blood pressure (Hamilton et al. 1983; Wenger and Stern 1983). In several large studies of depressed patients treated with bupropion, either small decreases (1–3 mm Hg) or no change in supine and standing systolic and diastolic blood pressure was observed (Chouinard et al. 1981; Hamilton et al. 1983; Remick et al. 1982; Wenger and Stern 1983). Nine of 12 patients previously exhibiting pronounced orthostatic hypotension during treatment with TCAs were successfully given therapeutic doses of bupropion without recurrence of clinically significant orthostasis (Farid et al. 1983).

In addition, the incidence of electrocardiographic abnormalities has not been different in bupropion and placebo-treated patients (Remick et al. 1982; Wenger and Stern 1983; Wenger et al. 1983), and the PR and QRS intervals are reported to be unchanged with bupropion treatment (Wenger and Stern 1983; Wenger et al. 1983). Five patients who overdosed on bupropion, 900 to 3,000 mg, had no serious cardiovascular changes (Wenger and Stern 1983).

Roose et al. (1987a) treated 10 depressed cardiac patients for 3 weeks each with both imipramine (3.5 kg/day at full dose) and bupropion (450 mg/day at full dose) in a crossover study. They found no adverse effect of either agent on the left ventricular ejection fraction, but the mean orthostatic systolic blood pressure drop was found to be 15 mm Hg on imipramine compared with only 2 mm Hg on bupropion. Five of the 10 patients developed orthostatic hypotension when treated with imipramine and none when treated with bupropion.

In summary, bupropion appears to offer a distinctly advantageous cardiovascular profile for treating the elderly depressed patient or those patients with cardiac disease.

Fluoxetine

Fluoxetine is a straight-chain phenylpropylamide that is structurally unrelated to the TCAs. In common with some of the TCAs, fluoxetine inhibits neuronal uptake of serotonin, but it has no effect on norepinephrine uptake and has little anticholinergic activity (Wong et al. 1975). Fluoxetine is metabolized to N-desmethyl fluoxetine, which is pharmacologically active, has a prolonged elimination half-life, and is also a selective inhibitor of serotonin uptake (Fuller et al. 1978).

Animal studies indicate that fluoxetine has few hemodynamic or electrophysiological effects, even in supratherapeutic doses (Benfield et al. 1986; Wernicke 1985). For example, Steinberg et al. (1986) administered fluoxetine, 0.1 mg/kg/min for 50 minutes, in anesthetized dogs and observed no significant reduction in heart rate, blood pressure, or pulmonary wedge pressure compared to a control group. Fluoxetine had no effect on cardiac conduction velocity as assessed by either surface or intracardiac conduction indices. In contrast, an infusion of amitriptyline at the same dose increased heart rate and reduced both mean arterial pressure and systemic vascular resistance. Amitriptyline also increased pulmonary wedge pressure and reduced stroke volume, suggesting impaired ventricular contractility. Importantly, amitriptyline also produced the expected delay in intraventricular conduction that was evidenced by prolongation of the PQ interval (interval from the beginning of the P wave to the start of the QRS complex) and QRS interval on the surface ECG and by lengthening of the HV interval (Purkinje fiber transmission) on the intracardiac recordings.

Findings from clinical studies of patients treated with fluoxetine parallel the findings from the animal studies. In therapeutic doses, fluoxetine treatment is associated with a small reduction in heart rate, but significant changes in blood pressure, electrocardiographic changes, and evidence of conduction delay do not occur (Benfield et al. 1986; Fisch 1985; Upward et al. 1988; Wernicke 1985).

Findings from both animal and human studies suggest that fluoxetine produces no clinically important cardiovascular effects at therapeutically effective doses. It is important to emphasize, however, that few human studies have been performed, and we are aware of no published data related to the cardiovascular effects of fluoxetine in patients selected for the presence of heart disease. Hopefully, such studies will be forthcoming and will confirm the promising outlook for this agent.

Cardiovascular Effects of Monoamine Oxidase Inhibitors, Psychostimulants, and Lithium

Monoamine Oxidase Inhibitors

In contrast to the TCAs, relatively few studies have investigated the cardiovascular effects of the MAO inhibitors. The cardiovascular profile of the MAO inhibitors differs from those of the TCAs, as might be expected given the differences in pharmacology of these two classes of drugs. In clinical studies, phenelzine treatment *reduces* heart rate and *shortens* the QT_c interval (Davidson and Turnbull 1986; Georgotas et al. 1987b; Robinson et al. 1981, 1982; White et al. 1983). An MAO inhibitor–induced increase in local norepinephrine availability at brain-stem $alpha_2$ receptors that inhibit sympathetic nervous system outflow and stimulate the motor nerve of the vagus (Isaac 1980; Veith et al. 1984) is a possible mechanism to explain the simultaneous reduction in blood pressure and decrease in heart rate that are associated with MAO inhibitor treatment.

An important clinical advantage of the MAO inhibitors for patients with conduction disturbances is the absence of an effect to delay intraventricular conduction (Georgotas et al. 1987a, 1987b; Goldman et al. 1986; McGrath et al. 1987; Robinson et al. 1981, 1982; White et al. 1983). Rare reports of rhythm disturbances associated with MAO inhibitor use have been described (White et al. 1983), but it does not appear that this class of antidepressant medications has any significant influence on cardiac rhythm. To our knowledge, the effect, if any, of the MAO inhibitors on myocardial performance has not yet been assessed in humans. However, we are aware of no evidence indicating a deleterious effect in elderly patients or in those patients with compromised ventricular function.

The MAO inhibitors have historically been used as antihypertensive agents. Not surprisingly, the most frequent serious cardiovascular effect of MAO inhibitor therapy is orthostatic hypotension (Davidson and Turnbull 1986; Georgotas et al. 1987a; Goldman et al. 1986; Kronig et al. 1983; Mallinger et al. 1986; Rabkin et al. 1985; Razani et al. 1983; Robinson et al. 1981, 1982). Although some studies suggest that the hypotensive effects of the MAO inhibitors are dose-related and correlated with plasma concentrations (Mallinger et al. 1986), this is not a consistent finding (Davidson and Turnbull 1986). It has also been reported that the maximal decrease in supine and orthostatic blood pressure may not occur until several weeks after initiating therapy (Feighner et al. 1985).

In addition to the hypotensive effects of MAO inhibitor therapy, the potential for hypertensive crisis in response to ingestion of tyramine-containing foods or sympathomimetic drugs is a serious concern. Rabkin et al. (1985) reported hypertensive reactions in 8% of their patients receiving phenelzine and 2% of those taking tranylcypromine. Obviously, patient education is critical in minimizing the risk of this serious adverse effect.

Psychostimulants

Psychostimulant medications (e.g., dexamphetamine, methylphenidate, magnesium pemoline) have a limited role in the pharmacology of psychiatric disorders (Chiarello and Cole 1987) but have acquired a selective popularity in the management of frail elderly patients (Katon and Raskind 1980; Satel and Nelson 1989). It is interesting that the popularity of the psychostimulants as an alternative strategy in the pharmacological treatment of depression has been sustained over the years because, as was recently reviewed by Satel and Nelson (1989), only 1 of 10 controlled trials has demonstrated superior efficacy compared with placebo. Although the efficacy of these agents is suspect, at least the psychostimulants appear to offer few hazards for the older patient.

The psychostimulants have the potential to elevate blood pressure, heart rate, and plasma catecholamine levels when given intravenously, but the sympathomimetic responses are modest when these agents are administered orally to normal subjects or depressed patients (Goldstein et al. 1983; Janowsky et al. 1978a, 1978b; Joyce et al. 1984; Nurnberger et al. 1984). The cardiovascular effects of orally administered psychostimulants have been described in numerous anecdotal clinical reports but have not been extensively investigated in elderly or medically ill patients. Crook et al. (1977) orally administered doses of 10 mg and 30 mg of methylphenidate to 12 elderly subjects with a mean age of 72 years and observed no changes in heart rate or blood pressure during the 90 minutes following ingestion. Two of eight subjects who were administered 45 mg orally had an increase in heart rate and blood pressure.

In summary, the psychostimulants should be relegated to a secondary role in the treatment of elderly patients. Anecdotal evidence suggests that the frail elderly patient who is unresponsive to or unable to tolerate traditional antidepressant therapy may benefit from a time-limited trial of a psychostimulant as an alternative strategy. In the usual doses in which they are employed to treat elderly depressed patients (i.e., 10–30 mg/day dexamphetamine or methylphenidate), the psychostimulants produce few significant cardiovascular effects (see Satel and Nelson 1989 for review).

Lithium

Lithium treatment is frequently associated with benign, nonspecific T-wave alterations on the ECG that are thought to reflect changes in myocardial repolarization at the cellular level. Of more serious concern, however, is lithium's potential to produce bradycardia by antagonizing sinus node function. As noted by Roose et al. (1979), this can occur within therapeutic lithium concentrations in subjects who are otherwise asymptomatic. For this reason, it is important to identify patients with occult sinus-node arrhythmias or "sick sinus syndrome" by routinely obtaining an ECG prior to initiating lithium treatment in older individuals.

Treatment Strategies for Treating the Elderly Patient

The primary task of the clinician considering antidepressant therapy for the older or medically ill patient is to ensure that the affective disturbance to be treated is of sufficient severity and duration to be considered qualitatively appropriate for pharmacological treatment. However, issues related to the diagnosis and differential diagnosis of major depression in this setting are beyond the scope of this review.

Prior to initiating antidepressant therapy, all elderly patients should be carefully evaluated for the presence of cardiac disease or other clinical risk factors that might predispose them to complications related to the antidepressant medications. Particular emphasis should be directed toward identifying patients with pretreatment orthostatic hypotension, congestive heart failure, and/or conduction disturbances.

The workup should include a careful history, a physical examination, and a 12-lead ECG. Pretreatment postural blood pressure measurements should also be assessed to serve as a baseline prior to instituting pharmacological treatment. Related physical or clinical factors that would be expected to increase the risks of cardiovascular complications include unstable medical or cardiac status (e.g., recent myocardial infarction, congestive heart failure, poorly controlled hypertension); deconditioning due to prolonged bed rest; concurrent use of medications that lower blood pressure or other agents that might interact with the antidepressants (e.g., anticholinergic drugs, class 1 antiarrhythmics); or sympathetic nervous system dysfunction (e.g., diabetes, Shy-Drager syndrome). Ideally, the patient's medical condition will have been stabilized and concurrent medication use will have been reduced as much as possible before instituting antidepressant treatment.

As noted above, two main concerns represent the major risks of antidepressant treatment in the elderly or medically ill patient: 1) the potential for many of these drugs to delay intraventricular conduction, and 2) the propensity of these agents to produce postural hypotension. From the narrow perspective of considering only the cardiovascular aspects of the antidepressants, it is possible to make several treatment recommendations for managing the elderly depressed patent. Obviously, the primary goal is to minimize risk while pursuing therapeutic efficacy. Therefore, we offer the following general guidelines.

Of the first-generation TCAs, evidence clearly favors the use of nortriptyline for the older patient with no known increased risk for conduction delay or postural hypotension. This agent 1) is relatively less anticholinergic than many of the original TCAs, 2) is effective in lower doses and plasma concentrations, 3) has been shown to produce fewer problems with orthostasis at those lower plasma levels, and 4) has the additional advantage of having a generally accepted optimal plasma concentration for efficacy (between 50–150 ng/ml). Unlike the newer agents, with which we do not yet have widespread clinical experience, nortriptyline has an established record of efficacy and safety, and thus it represents a reasonable first choice for the majority of elderly patients.

Several circumstances might dictate an alternative selection. The first is the possibility that this agent is proven to be ineffective or that its less prominent, but not insignificant, anticholinergic or blood pressure effects cannot be tolerated, requiring a switch to another agent. Of more concern are the patients with significant pretreatment orthostatic hypotension or congestive heart failure who appear to be at the greatest risk of the TCAs causing serious blood pressure complications. Finally, the presence of clinically significant conduction disturbances (i.e., bundle branch block, fascicular block, 2:1 atrioventricular block) prior to treatment or the development of these abnormalities during treatment may preclude nortriptyline treatment. In these situations, several possible strategies could be entertained.

The MAO inhibitors do not delay intracardiac conduction and could be considered when conduction disturbances are a concern. However, the potential for orthostatic hypotension is a risk that could potentially eliminate this alternative for many patients. The alternative, of course, is to consider the use of either bupropion or fluoxetine, both of which appear to be devoid of significant effects on cardiac conduction or blood pressure. Perhaps the only reason not to select these agents as first-choice drugs is that there is still limited experience with these agents on the national level, and for fluoxetine, there is little published information on how this agent is tolerated by individuals with serious cardiac disease. There are, of course, other issues to consider related to the noncardiovascular side-effect profiles of these newer agents, but that topic is not our primary focus in this review. It should also be noted in this context that electroconvulsive treatment is effective and well tolerated by elderly patients and should not be discounted as a treatment alternative.

After deciding upon the drug to be employed, several management issues should be kept in mind during the treatment course. A gradual dosage increment, starting at lower doses than might be used among young, healthy patients, is a useful technique to enhance compliance and to minimize adverse effects. Postural blood pressure should be monitored regularly. Depending upon the assessed risk of the patient, serial electrocardiographic monitoring should be considered for patients with a significant risk for conduction delay. Repeat ECGs should be obtained with an awareness of the elimination half-life of the agent employed.

For example, there is little reassurance gained by obtaining an ECG within less than a week after a dosing increment with nortriptyline, because at least that length of time will be required before steady-state plasma concentrations will be achieved. In this regard, it may require several weeks to achieve steady state with fluoxetine because of the prolonged half-life of its active metabolite. There is some benefit in obtaining an ECG after final steady-state doses of the antidepressants have been achieved for all older patients, primarily to document the electrocardiographic status of the patients at that point for future reference, in case a cardiac event ensues at a later point in treatment. It is also important to obtain a pretreatment ECG in older patients prior to instituting lithium treatment in order to identify individuals who might be predisposed to sinus node dysfunction.

References

Ahles S, Gwirtsman H, Halaris A, et al: Comparative cardiac effects of maprotiline and doxepin in elderly depressed patients. J Clin Psychiatry 45(11):460–465, 1984

Aronson MD, Hafez H: A case of trazodone-induced ventricular tachycardia. J Clin Psychiatry 47:388–389, 1986

Benfield P, Heck RC, Lewis SP: Fluoxetine: a review of its pharmacodynamic and pharmacokinetic properties, and therapeutic efficacy in depressive illness. Drugs 32:481–508, 1986

Bigger JT Jr, Giardina EGV, Perel JM, et al: Cardiac antiarrhythmic effect of imipramine hydrochloride. N Engl J Med 296:206–208, 1977

Boehnert MT, Lovejoy FJ Jr: Value of the QRS duration versus the serum drug level in predicting seizures and ventricular arrhythmias after an acute overdose of tricyclic antidepressants. N Engl J Med 313:474–479, 1985

Brorson L, Wennerblom B: Effect of the tetracyclic antidepressant drug maprotiline on cardiac electrophysiology in human volunteers. J Cardiovasc Pharmacol 4:531–535, 1982

Burrows GD, Vohra J, Dumovic P, et al: TCA drugs and cardiac conduction. Prog Neuropsychopharmacol 1:329–334, 1977

Byrne JE, Gomoll AW: Differential effects of trazodone and imipramine on intracardiac conduction in the anesthetized dog. Arch Int Pharmacodyn Ther 259:259–270, 1982

Charalampous KD: Amoxapine: a clinical evaluation in depressive symptoms. Current Therapeutic Research 14:657–663, 1972

Chiarello RJ, Cole JO: The use of psychostimulants in general psychiatry: a reconsideration. Arch Gen Psychiatry 44:286–295, 1987

Chouinard G, Annable L, Langlois R: Absence of orthostatic hypotension in depressed patients treated with bupropion. Prog Neuropsychopharmacol 5:483–490, 1981

Clements-Jewry S, Robson PA, Chidley LJ: Biochemical investigations into the mode of action of trazodone. Neuropharmacology 19:1165–1173, 1980

Connolly S, Mitchell L, Swerdlow C, et al: Clinical efficacy and electrophysiology of imipramine for ventricular tachycardia. Am J Cardiol 53:516–521, 1984

Coupet J, Rauh CE, Szues-Myers VA, et al: 2-Chloro-11-(1-piperazinyl)-dibenz[b,f] [1,4]oxazepine (amoxapine), an antidepressant with antipsychotic properties: a possible role for 7-hydroxyamoxapine. Biochem Pharmacol 28:2514–2515, 1979

Crook T, Ferris S, Sathananthan G, et al: The effect of methylphenidate on test performance in the congnitively impaired aged. Psychopharmacolgy (Berlin) 52:251–255, 1977

Davidson J, Turnbull CD: The effects of isocarboxazid on blood pressure and pulse. J Clin Psychopharmacol 6:139–143, 1986

Edwards JG, Goldie A: Mianserin, maprotiline and intracardiac conduction. Br J Clin Pharmacol 15:249S–254S, 1983

Farid FF, Wenger TL, Tsai SY, et al: Use of bupropion in patients who exhibit orthostatic hypotension on tricyclic antidepressants. J Clin Psychiatry 44 (5, sec 2):170–173, 1983

Feighner JP, Herbstein J, Damlouji N: Combined MAOI, TCA, and direct stimulant therapy of treatment-resistant depression. J Clin Psychiatry 46(6):206–209, 1985

Ferns KM, White H, Russell A, et al: The effects of bupropion HCl on uptake of biogenic amines and on inhibition of MAO. Federation Proceedings 37:481, 1978

Fisch C: Effect of fluoxetine on the electrocardiogram. J Clin Psychiatry 46 (3, sec 2):42–44, 1985

Foulke G, Albertson T: QRS interval in tricyclic antidepressant overdosage: inaccuracy as a toxicity indicator in emergency settings. Ann Emerg Med 16:160–163, 1987

Fuller RW, Snoddy HD, Perry KW, et al: Importance of duration of drug action in the antagonism of p-chloroamphetamine depletion of brain serotonin: comparison of fluoxetine and chlorimipramine. Biochem Pharmacol 27:193–198, 1978

Georgotas A, McCue RE, Friedman E, et al: Electrocardiographic effects of nortriptyline, phenelzine, and placebo under optimal treatment conditions. Am J Psychiatry 144:798–801, 1987a

Georgotas A, McCue RE, Friedman E, et al: A placebo-controlled comparison of the effect of nortriptyline and phenelzine on orthostatic hypotension in elderly depressed patients. J Clin Psychopharmacol 7:413–416, 1987b

Giardina EGV, Bigger JT Jr: Antiarrhythmic effect of imipramine hydrochloride in patients with ventricular premature complexes without psychological depression. Am J Cardiol 540:172–179, 1982

Giardina EGV, Barnard T, Johnson L, et al: The antiarrhythmic effect of nortriptyline in cardiac patients with ventricular premature depolarization. J Am Coll Cardiol 7:1363–1369, 1986

Giardina EGV, Cooper TB, Suckow R, et al: Cardiovascular effects of doxepin in cardiac patients with ventricular arrhythmias. Clin Pharmacol Ther 42:20–27, 1987

Glassman AH, Bigger JT Jr: Cardiovascular effects of therapeutic doses of tricyclic antidepressants. Arch Gen Psychiatry 38:815–820, 1981

Glassman AH, Bigger JT Jr, Giardina EGV, et al: Clinical characteristics of imipramine-induced orthostatic hypotension. Lancet 1:468–472, 1979

Glassman AH, Johnson LL, Giardina EGV, et al: The use of imipramine in depressed patients with congestive heart failure. JAMA 250:1997–2001, 1983

Goldberg RJ, Capone RJ, Hunt JD: Cardiac complications following tricyclic antidepressant overdose: issues for monitoring policy. JAMA 254:1772–1775, 1985

Goldman LS, Alexander RC, Luchins DJ: Monoamine oxidase inhibitors and tricyclic antidepressants: comparison of their cardiovascular effects. J Clin Psychiatry 47(5):225–229, 1986

Goldstein DS, Nurnberger J Jr, Simmons S, et al: Effects of injected sympathomimetic amines on plasma catecholamines and circulatory variables in man. Life Sci 32:1057–1063, 1983

Gomoll AW, Byrne JE, Deitchman D: Hemodynamic and cardiac actions of trazodone and imipramine in the anesthetized dog. Life Sci 24:1841–1848, 1979

Greenblatt EN, Lippa AS, Osterberg AC: The neuropharmacological actions of amoxapine. Arch Int Pharmacodyn 233:107–135, 1978

Hames TK, Burgess CD, George CF: Hemodynamic responses to trazodone and imipramine. Clin Pharmacol Ther 26:497–502, 1982

Hamilton MJ, Smith PR, Peck AW: Effects of bupropion, nomifensine and dexamphetamine on performance, subjective feelings, autonomic variables and electroencephalogram in healthy volunteers. Br J Clin Pharmacol 15:367–374, 1983

Hayes RL, Gerner RH, Fairbanks L, et al: ECG findings in geriatric depressives given trazodone, placebo, or imipramine. J Clin Psychiatry 44(5):180–183, 1983

Henry JA, Ali CJ, Caldwell R, et al: Acute trazodone poisoning: clinical signs and plasma concentrations. Psychopathology 17 (suppl 2):71–81, 1984

Hertzman M, Goins R: Amoxapine and heart disease (letter). J Clin Psychopharmacol 4:59–61, 1984

Himmelhoch JM: Cardiovascular effects of trazodone in humans. J Clin Psychopharmacol 1 (suppl):76S–81S, 1981

Himmelhoch JM, Schechtmen K, Auerbach R: The role of trazodone in the treatment of depressed cardiac patients. Psychopathology 17 (suppl 2):51–63, 1984

Irwin M, Spar JE: Reversible cardiac conduction abnormality associated with trazodone administration (letter). Am J Psychiatry 140:945–946, 1983

Isaac L: Clonidine in the central nervous system: site and mechanism of hypotensive action. J Cardiovasc Pharmacol 2:S5–S19, 1980

Janowsky DS, Leichner P, Parker D, et al: The effect of methylphenidate on serum growth hormone: influence of antipsychotic drugs and diagnosis. Arch Gen Psychiatry 35:1384–1389, 1978a

Janowsky DS, Leichner P, Parker D, et al: Methylphenidate and serum prolactin in man. Psychopharmacology (Berlin) 58:43–57, 1978b

Janowsky D, Curtis G, Zisook S, et al: Ventricular arrhythmias possibly aggravated by trazodone. Am J Psychiatry 140:796–797, 1983

Joyce PR, Nicholls MG, Donald RA: Methylphenidate increases heart rate, blood pressure, and plasma epinephrine in normal subjects. Life Sci 34:1707–1711, 1984

Kantor SJ, Bigger JT Jr, Glassman AH, et al: Imipramine-induced heart block: a longitudinal case study. JAMA 231:1364–1366, 1975

Katon W, Raskind MA: Treatment of depression in the medically ill elderly with methylphenidate. Am J Psychiatry 137:963–965, 1980

Kronig MH, Roose SP, Walsh BT, et al: Blood pressure effects of phenelzine. J Clin Psychopharmacol 3:307–310, 1983

Kulig K, Rumack BH, Sullivan JB, et al: Amoxapine overdose: coma and seizures without cardiovascular effects. JAMA 248:1092–1094, 1982

Langou RA, Van Dyke C, Tahan SR, et al: Cardiovascular manifestations of tricyclic antidepressant overdose. Am Heart J 100:458–464, 1980

Leighton HJ, Maxwell RA: The autonomic and cardiovascular pharmacology of bupropion HCl. Federation Proceedings 37:481, 1978

Lindbom L-O, Groschinsky-Grind M, Forsberg T: Comparative cardiovascular effects of antidepressants in animals and man. J Clin Psychiatry 43(5, sec 2):32–34, 1982

Lippmann SB: Trazodone cardiac effects. International Drug Therapy Newsletter 20:29–32, 1985

Lisciani R, Baldini A, Benedetti D, et al: Acute cardiovascular toxicity of trazodone, etoperidone and imipramine in rats. Toxicology 10:151–158, 1978

Litovitz JL, Troutman WG: Amoxapine overdose: seizures and fatalities. JAMA 250:1069–1071, 1983

Luchins DJ: Review of clinical and animal studies comparing the cardiovascular effects of doxepin and other tricyclic antidepressants. Am J Psychiatry 140:1006–1009, 1983

Maj J, Palider W, Rawlow A: Trazodone, a central serotonin antagonist. J Neural Transm 44:237–248, 1979

Mallinger AG, Edwards DJ, Himmelhoch JM, et al: Pharmacokinetics of tranylcypromine in patients who are depressed: relationship to cardiovascular effects. Clin Pharmacol Ther 40:444–450, 1986

McGrath PJ, Blood DK, Stewart JW, et al: A comparative study of the electrocardiographic effects of phenelzine, tricyclic antidepressants, mianserin, and placebo. J Clin Psychopharmacol 7:335–339, 1987

Moriarty RW: Tricyclic antidepressant poisoning. Drug Therapy (Hospital Edition) 6:73–82, 1981

Muir WW, Strauch SM, Schaal SF: Effects of tricyclic antidepressant drugs on the electrophysiological properties of dog Purkinje fibers. J Cardiovasc Pharmacol 4:82–90, 1982

Nelson JC, Jatlow PI, Mazure C: Desipramine plasma levels and response in elderly melancholic patients. J Clin Psychopharmacol 5:217–220, 1985

Nurnberger JI, Simmons-Alling S, Kessler L, et al: Separate mechanisms for behavioral, cardiovascular, and hormonal responses to dextroamphetamine in man. Psychopharmacology (Berlin) 84:200–204, 1984

Pumariega AJ, Muller B, Rivers-Bulkeley N: Acute renal failure secondary to amoxapine overdose. JAMA 248:3141–3142, 1982

Rabkin JG, Quitkin FM, McGrath P, et al: Adverse reactions to monoamine oxidase inhibitors, Part II: treatment correlates and clinical management. J Clin Psychopharmacol 5:2–9, 1985

Raeder EA, Zinsli M, Burckhardt D: Effect of maprotiline on cardiac arrhythmias. Br Med J 2:102, 1979

Rausch J, Pavlinac DM, Newman PE: Complete heart block following a single dose of trazodone. Am J Psychiatry 141:1472–1473, 1984

Razani J, White KL, White J, et al: The safety and efficacy of combined amitriptyline and tranylcypromine antidepressant treatment: a controlled trial. Arch Gen Psychiatry 40:657–661, 1983

Reis DJ, Morrison S, Ruggiero DA: The C1 area of the brain stem in tonic and reflex control of blood pressure: state-of-the-art lecture. Hypertension 11 (suppl 1):8–13, 1988

Remick RA, Campos PE, Misri S, et al: A comparison of the safety and efficacy of bupropion HCl and amitriptyline HCl in depressed outpatients. Prog Neuropsychopharmacol Biol Psychiatry 6:523–527, 1982

Riblet LA, Gatewood CF, Mayol RF: Comparative effects of trazodone and tricyclic antidepressants on uptake of selected neurotransmitters by isolated brain synaptosomes. Psychopharmacology (Berlin) 63:99–101, 1979

Richelson E: The newer antidepressants: structures, pharmacodynamics, and proposed mechanisms of action. Psychopharmacol Bull 20:213–223, 1984

Robinson DS, Corcella J, Nies A, et al: Cardiovascular effects of amitriptyline and phenelzine. Clin Pharmacol Ther 29:276–277, 1981

Robinson DS, Nies A, Corcella J, et al: Cardiovascular effects of phenelzine and amitriptyline in depressed outpatients. J Clin Psychiatry 43 (5, sec 2):8–15, 1982

Robinson DS, Corcella J, Feighner JP, et al: A comparison of trazodone, amoxapine and maprotiline in the treatment of endogenous depression: results of a multicenter study. Current Therapeutic Research 35:549–560, 1984

Roose SP, Nurnberger JI, Dunner DL, et al: Cardiac sinus node dysfunction during lithium treatment. Am J Psychiatry 136:804–806, 1979

Roose SP, Glassman AH, Siris SG, et al: Comparison of imipramine- and nortriptyline-induced orthostatic hypotension: a meaningful difference. J Clin Psychopharmacol 1:316–319, 1981

Roose SP, Glassman AH, Giardina EGV, et al: Nortriptyline in depressed patients with left ventricular impairment. JAMA 256:3253–3257, 1986

Roose SP, Glassman AH, Giardina EGV, et al: Cardiovascular effects of imipramine and bupropion in depressed patients with congestive heart failure. J Clin Psychopharmacol 7:247–251, 1987a

Roose SP, Glassman AH, Giardina EGV, et al: Tricyclic antidepressants in depressed patients with cardiac conduction disease. Arch Gen Psychiatry 44:273–275, 1987b

Satel SL, Nelson JC: Stimulants in the treatment of depression: a critical overview. J Clin Psychiatry 50(7):241–249, 1989

Sawchenko PE, Cunningham ET, Levin MC: Anatomic and biochemical specificity in central autonomic pathways, in Organization of the Autonomic Nervous System: Central and Peripheral Mechanisms. Edited by Cirello J. New York, AR Liss, 1987, pp 267–281

Silverberg AB, Shah SD, Haymond MW, et al: Norepinephrine: hormone and neurotransmitter in man. Am J Physiol 234:E252–E256, 1978

Smith RB, Rusbatch BJ: Amitriptyline and heart block. Br Med J 3:311, 1967

Soroko FE, Maxwell RA: The pharmacologic basis for therapeutic interest in bupropion. J Clin Psychiatry 44 (5, sec 2):67–73, 1983

Spiker DB, Weiss AN, Chang SS, et al: Tricyclic antidepressant overdose: clinical presentation and plasma levels. Clin Pharmacol Ther 18:539–546, 1975

Steinberg MI, Smallwood JK, Holland DR, et al: Hemodynamic and electrocardiographic effects of fluoxetine and its major metabolite, norfluoxetine, in anesthetized dogs. Toxicol Appl Pharmacol 82:70–79, 1986

Stoudemire A, Atkinson P: Use of cyclic antidepressants in patients with cardiac conduction disturbances. Gen Hosp Psychiatry 10:389–397, 1988

Thayssen P, Bjerre M, Kragh-Sorensen P, et al: Cardiovascular effects of imipramine in elderly patients. Psychopharmacology (Berlin) 74:360–364, 1981

Upward JW, Edwards JG, Goldie A, et al: Comparative effects of fluoxetine and amitriptyline on cardiac function. Br J Clin Pharmacol 26:399–402, 1988

Veith RC, Bloom V, Bielski R, et al: ECG effects of comparable plasma concentrations of desipramine and amitriptyline. J Clin Psychopharmacol 2:394–398, 1982a

Veith RC, Raskind MA, Caldwell JH, et al: Cardiovascular effects of tricyclic antidepressants. N Engl J Med 306:954–959, 1982b

Veith RC, Raskind MA, Barnes RF, et al: Tricyclic antidepressants and supine, standing, and exercise plasma norepinephrine levels. Clin Pharmacol Ther 33:763–769, 1983

Veith RC, Best JD, Halter JB: Dose-dependent suppression of norepinephrine appearance rate in plasma by clonidine in man. J Clin Endocrinol Metab 59:151–155, 1984

Vlay SC, Friedling S: Trazodone exacerbation of V.T. (letter). Am Heart J 106:604, 1983

Weld FM, Bigger JT Jr: Electrophysiological effects of imipramine on ovine cardiac Purkinje and ventricular muscle fibers. Circ Res 46:167–175, 1980

Wenger TL, Stern WC: The cardiovascular profile of bupropion. J Clin Psychiatry 44 (5, sec 2):176–182, 1983

Wenger TL, Cohn JB, Bustrack J: Comparison of the effects of bupropion and amitriptyline on cardiac conduction in depressed patients. J Clin Psychiatry 44(5, sec 2):174–175, 1983

Wernicke JF: The side effect profile and safety of fluoxetine. J Clin Psychiatry 46 (3, sec 2):59–67, 1985

White K, O'Leary J, Razani J, et al: Electrocardiographic effects of tranylcypromine vs amitriptyline. J Clin Psychiatry 44(3):91–93, 1983

White WB, Wong SHY: Rapid atrial fibrillation associated with trazodone hydrochloride. Arch Gen Psychiatry 42:424, 1985

Wilkerson RD: Antiarrhythmic effects of tricyclic antidepressant drugs in ouabain-induced arrhythmias in the dog. J Pharmacol Exp Ther 205:666–674, 1978

Wong DT, Horng JS, Bymaster FP, et al: A new selective inhibitor for uptake of serotonin into synaptosomes of rat brain: 3-(p-tri-fluoromethylphenoxy)-N-methyl-3-phenylpropylamine. J Pharmacol Exp Ther 193:804–811, 1975

Zavodnick S: Atrial flutter with amoxapine: a case report. Am J Psychiatry 138:1503–1504, 1981

Chapter 3

Neurological Side Effects of Psychotropic Medications in the Elderly

Larry E. Tune, M.D.

*P*sychotropic medications are commonly administered to manage the behavioral manifestations of dementing illness. It is clear, however, based on extensive experience, that toxicity from psychotropic medications themselves poses a serious challenge to the clinician. In the following review, toxicity from neuroleptic and anticholinergic medications will be extensively examined.

Neuroleptic Toxicity

Review of the Literature

Symptoms of dementia include a variety of distressing behavioral disturbances ranging from mild irritability and sleeplessness to episodic violence, delusions, and hallucinations. The management of these symptoms presents a major challenge to practitioners in the community and in long-term care facilities. Neuroleptic medications have been the mainstay of treatment of these behavioral symptoms in the elderly.

A number of studies evaluating the use of neuroleptics have been reported. We reviewed 29 studies involving the use of neuroleptics in various elderly, demented groups (for detailed review, see Tune et al. 1991). Twenty-seven of these studies showed distinct clinical improvement in behaviors ranging from agitation and hyperactivity to delusions and hallucinations. One (Cahn and Diesfeldt 1973) showed no improvement over placebo in a double-blind study of penfluridol. Gotestam et al.

(1981) found that haloperidol (0.5–1.0 mg/day) resulted in "significant clinical deterioration." Twenty-three of 29 studies reported on side effects, particularly extrapyramidal side effects and sedation/lethargy. In all studies, neuroleptic side effects posed a significant problem to the clinical management of the patient. Most of these studies were of short duration, with little consideration given to prevalence and significance of side effects occurring with chronic use. Because Alzheimer's disease is the most common dementing illness, and because behavioral symptoms are common and troublesome in the care of patients with this disease throughout the course of illness, evaluation of neuroleptic therapy and the development of guidelines for the use of neuroleptics in this particular type of dementia are important.

In a prior study (Steele et al. 1986), we compared the use of haloperidol and thioridazine in the behavioral management of 17 patients with senile dementia of the Alzheimer type (SDAT). Both drugs were effective in managing targeted behavioral symptoms, but the side-effect profiles appeared to be different. Extrapyramidal side effects were present in all patients receiving ≥ 2 mg haloperidol per day. By contrast, only 8 of 16 subjects had extrapyramidal side effects on 75 mg per day of thioridazine.

In a follow-up study, summarized below, these two commonly prescribed neuroleptics, haloperidol and thioridazine, were evaluated in a double-blind protocol.

Side-Effect Profile Study

Methods and patient population.   Thirty-one patients who satisfied DSM-III-R criteria (American Psychiatric Association 1987) for primary degenerative dementia and NINCDS-ADRDA criteria (McKhann et al. 1984) for probable SDAT were studied. Eighteen were female and 13 were male. The average age of the sample was 68.2 years ± 1.14 SEM. Ten patients were residents of a nursing home facility, and the remaining 21 were outpatients enrolled in the Dementia Research Clinic (DRC) of the Johns Hopkins Hospital for both diagnosis and management of dementing illness. All outpatients were examined in the DRC and had appropriate laboratory tests to screen for treatable causes of dementia (i.e., SMA-6, SMA-12, HEME-8, B_{12}, folate, thyroid function tests). All received a computed tomography (CT) scan and electroencephalographic assessment as part of the diagnostic workup.

All patients were screened using the Sandoz Clinical Assessment Scale for Geriatric Symptoms (SCAG) (Shader et al. 1974). This 18-item questionnaire rates a variety of behavioral symptoms common in patients with dementing illness. Each symptom is rated for severity on a scale of 0 to 8. To be included in the project, all patients must have had at least one significant behavioral symptom that received a score of 4 or more, indicating moderately severe psychopathology. In the clinical evaluation of each patient by a research physician (L.E.T.), symptoms identified were of sufficient severity to necessitate neuroleptic treatment.

Study medications were formulated in identical capsules, and medications were administered according to a randomization scheme. Investigators, subjects, family, caregivers, and, in the case of the institutionalized patients, the nursing staff, were all blind to the drug assignment of the subjects. If subjects were previously taking any sychotropic medications, the medications were discontinued for a 2-week wash-out period before entry into the study. In three instances, after the wash-out period, the subjects' behavioral disturbances resolved and these individuals were excluded from the study. It was possible that the disturbances were related to delirium for those previously prescribed medications.

Clinical design.   Once entered, incremental doses of either thioridazine or haloperidol were given. Doses of thioridazine were 12.5, 25.0, 37.5, 50.0, 67.5, and 75.0 mg per day. Doses of haloperidol were 0.5, 1.0, 1.5, 2.0, 2.5, and 3.0 mg per day. All patients remained on a given dose for 2 weeks. Dosage increments occurred following clinical examination by the investigators. The following rating instruments were administered: SCAG (Shader et al. 1974); the Mini-Mental State Examination (MMSE) (Folstein et al. 1975); vital signs, including orthostatic blood pressures; and the DiMascio Rating Scale for Extrapyramidal Symptoms (DiMascio et al. 1976).

At each clinical evaluation, one of three decisions was made: 1) to increase dose when sufficient clinical improvement had not been achieved, 2) to continue at current dose when adequate response was seen, or 3) to drop the patient from the study because of significant side effects. Clinical improvement was defined a priori as a 2-point improvement on the SCAG score for the targeted behaviors. Significant side effects were considered to be 1) the presence of delirium, diagnosed clinically and supported by a decrease of at least 2 points in the MMSE score; 2) the presence of orthostatic hypotension as demonstrated by orthostatic changes in blood pressure associated with the presence of clinical symptoms (e.g., dizziness); or 3) the presence of significant extrapyramidal side effects as demonstrated by a score of 3 or more on the DiMascio scale.

If the patient did not show a significant improvement in behavioral symptoms and did not show significant side effects, the next dosage increment was initiated. If the patient demonstrated significant side effects, he or she was immediately dropped from the study. If the patient showed clinical improvement and did not demonstrate significant side effects, then he or she was enrolled in a continuation phase of the study, in which his or her current dose of neuroleptic medication was maintained for a period of 3 months. Reassessments in the continuation phase were conducted at 3 months using the aforementioned rating instruments.

Results.   As Figures 3-1 and 3-2 indicate, only three patients completed the entire study (including stabilization phase) without developing significant side effects. Two of these received thioridazine and one received haloperidol. None of the patients developed orthostatic hypotension. Patients were dropped from the study primarily for extreme drowsiness ($n = 7$) or parkinsonian symptoms ($n = 5$). Four patients were dropped during the study because of noncompliance. However, on review of the records, this noncompliance was very likely due to the onset of side effects during the study. One patient developed "dizzy spells" with a pulse of less than 60. There was no clear evidence of orthostatic changes on any examination. One patient died from unrelated causes while in the study.

Fifteen of the patients studied initially were entered into the stabilization phase. They demonstrated significant clinical improvement in the absence of significant side effects on initial examination. Side effects emerged during the subsequent 3 months of stabilization. Of the 15 patients entered into the stabilization phase, 7 developed significant side effects. Of the remaining 8 patients, all showed some evidence of drug toxicity but did not satisfy the exclusionary criteria articulated in the methods section above. Three became mildly confused, and 5 developed mild parkinsonian symptoms. Most of these side effects occurred with haloperidol (see Figure 3-1) during the last 6 weeks of the stabilization phase.

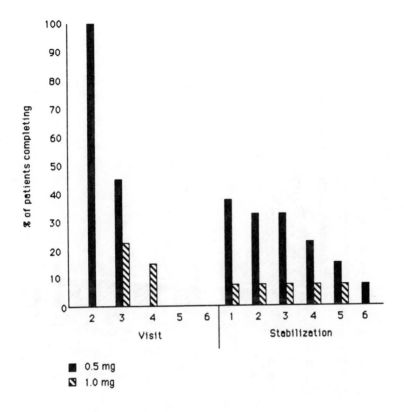

Figure 3–1.   Occurrence of haloperidol-induced side effects, expressed as a percentage of patients at various stages of the protocol. Patients (*n* = 13) received escalating doses of haloperidol. Haloperidol doses were 0.5 mg (black bars) and 1.0 mg (hatched bars) per day. Only one patient (0.5 mg/day) completed the study without side effects.

Discussion

Physicians have long been wary of chronically administering neuroleptic medications to the demented elderly for fear of significant side effects. These fears are supported by our data. Surprisingly, only one patient developed significant problems that may have been related to orthostasis. Two other patients developed cardiac symptoms in the form of decreased pulse rate. Haloperidol and thioridazine were equally problematic regard-

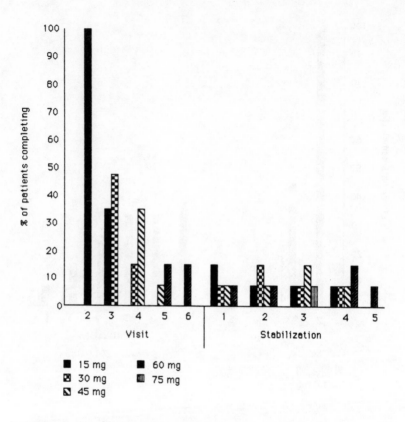

Figure 3–2. Occurrence of thioridazine-induced side effects, expressed as a percentage of patients at various stages of the protocol. Patients ($n = 15$) received escalating doses of thioridazine. Two patients completed the study without side effects; both received 60 mg per day of thioridazine.

ing patients developing significant extrapyramidal symptoms. Given thioridazine's inherent anticholinergic effects, we expected that patients would develop fewer extrapyramidal symptoms on this medication. However, as our own group has demonstrated, the doses of thioridazine utilized in this particular protocol rarely demonstrate significant anticholinergic effects as evidenced by serum anticholinergic levels (Steele et al. 1986). Both drugs were equally efficacious in managing behavioral symptoms and bore the same liability in terms of significant side effects.

One major contribution of this study, however, is the demonstration of late-emerging side effects. Patients who were successfully treated with low doses of either haloperidol or thioridazine developed significant side effects several months after the treatment dose was established. At least 7 out of 18 patients developed these symptoms in the first 3 months of the stabilization dose. This finding could be related to such factors as the progressive nature of the underlying disease process, accumulation of the neuroleptic over time, or receptor supersensitivity secondary to chronic stimulation from the neuroleptic. It is therefore prudent to monitor patients frequently, at least for the first 3 months after the treatment dose is established.

Anticholinergic Toxicity

Elderly patients are at particular risk for developing toxicity from anticholinergic medications because of 1) age-related decline in cholinergic neurotransmission, and 2) concurrent medical illnesses requiring use (often chronically) of multiple medications, some of which have known anticholinergic effects, and many more of which have often unrecognized additive antagonistic effects on cholinergic neurotransmission (Lipowski 1990). The risk of delirium may increase as a function of increasing numbers of prescribed medications with anticholinergic effects. The potential size of this problem was illustrated by Blazer et al. (1983), who found that 60% of a sample of 5,902 nursing home residents and 23% of elderly control subjects received anticholinergic medications. As many as 10%–17% of nursing home patients received three or more anticholinergic medications in a single year; 5% of patients received five or more anticholinergic medications in a single year.

Work from our own group provides direct evidence for anticholinergic-induced delirium. We have measured anticholinergic drug levels using a radioreceptor assay method in a variety of patient groups. In order to evaluate the anticholinergic effects of parent compounds, pharmacologically active metabolites, and drug combinations, we modified an existing radioreceptor assay technique to assess the antimuscarinic anticholinergic effects of medications in human serum (Tune and Coyle 1981). The assay is based on the fact that the potent muscarinic antagonist [3H]quinuclidinyl benzilate ([3H]-QNB) binds specifically and avidly to muscarinic receptors. Drugs that block muscarinic receptors, regardless of structure, compete with [3H]-QNB binding at muscarinic receptors. Specific binding of QNB to muscarinic receptors is reduced in proportion to the concentration and potency of anticholinergic drugs in serum. Using this assay in a variety of clinical settings, we made the following observations.

1. Relationship between dose of a known anticholinergic medication and serum anticholinergic drug level. As Figures 3-3 and 3-4 demonstrate, there was substantial variability of anticholinergic drug level for compounds with anticholinergic properties. In particular, there was 1) at least a 10-fold variation in drug level at a given dose of the anticholinergic drug benztropine mesylate, 2) a poor correlation between dose and serum drug level, and 3) (what appears to be) nonlinear pharmacokinetics of anticholinergic drugs, in patients who are followed longitudinally. The relationship between the serum level of anticholinergic drugs and the total daily dose of benztropine mesylate in 49 patients is shown in Figure 3-3. A poor correlation was found between serum anticholinergic levels and total daily dose of benztropine mesylate. With doses of 2, 3, 4, and 6 mg/day, serum drug levels varied nearly 100-fold from the highest to the lowest level. The average serum levels for these different dosages were 17 pmol/ml atropine equivalents at 2 mg/day, 11 pmol at 3 mg/day, 12 pmol at 4 mg/day, and 27 pmol at 6 mg/day.

2. Anticholinergic drug levels and delirium. In a number of clinical settings, we have demonstrated significant correlations between elevated serum concentrations of anticholinergic medications (as measured by radioreceptor assays) and cognitive impairment, including delirium. In a study of patients undergoing open-heart cardiac surgery (Tune et al. 1981), 29 patients were screened pre- and postoperatively with the MMSE (Folstein et al. 1975) to assess general cognitive state. Patients were evaluated preoperatively, within 24 hours postoperatively, and up to three times a week for the subsequent 2 weeks. At the time of each evaluation, serum anticholinergic drug levels were obtained.

Ten of 29 (34.5%) patients became delirious during the first postoperative week. Twenty-five of these 29 patients were evaluated within the first 24 hours after surgery. Of these, 8 were delirious. Seven of the 8 patients who were delirious in the first 24 hours had significantly elevated serum anticholinergic drug levels (> 1.5 pmol/sample atropine equivalents). Only 4 of the nondelirious patients had serum anticholinergic drug concentrations above 1.5 pmol/sample ($X^2 = 11.53$, $P < .001$).

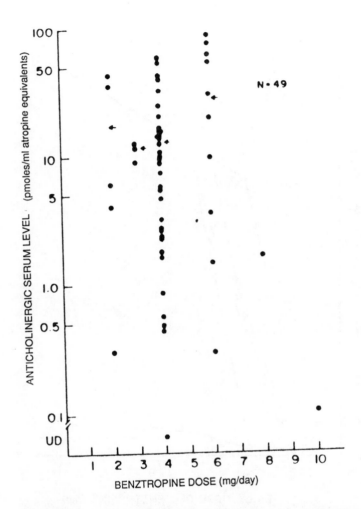

Figure 3–3. Serum samples were obtained from 49 inpatients who received a fixed dose of benztropine mesylate for at least 4 days prior to sample called on. Results for the radioreceptor assay are expressed in terms of the amount of atropine (pmol) that produced the same amount of inhibition as caused by the patient's serum and expressed as ml atropine equivalents. Arrows indicate mean drug level for each daily dose (Tune and Coyle 1981). Six patients were followed longitudinally with increasing orally administered dosage of benztropine mesylate. A nonlinear relationship between daily dose and serum anticholinergic level was observed (see Figure 3-4) in many cases.

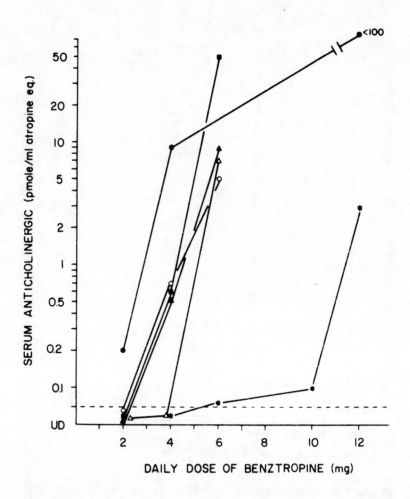

Figure 3–4. Six schizophrenic patients receiving benztropine mesylate for control of extrapyramidal side effects were evaluated longitudinally with serum anticholinergic drug levels following increasing doses of benztropine mesylate. Each line represents data from one patient (Tune and Coyle 1981). In some cases, slight (2-mg) increments in oral dose were associated with a several-fold increase in the serum concentration of anticholinergic activity.

The decline in MMSE scores was highly significantly correlated with serum anticholinergic level ($r = .83$, $n = 24$, $P < .001$) (Figure 3-5). As serum levels of anticholinergic drugs increased, there was a steady decline in cognitive functioning as assessed by a decline in MMSE scores compared with presurgery MMSE scores.

The 10 delirious patients were administered an average of 8 medications. Many of these medications, according to a scale devised by Summers (1978), are associated with delirium, and some have known anticholinergic effects. Patients who became delirious received an average of 4.0 drugs that were known to have been associated with delirium. The nondelirious patients received an average of 2.7 drugs. This differ-

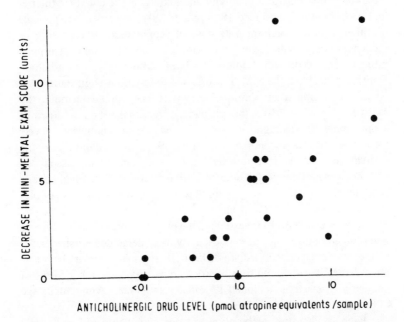

Figure 3–5. Change in Mini-Mental State Examination (MMSE) score in 29 patients undergoing open-heart surgery. Results are expressed as the decline in MMSE score between pre- and postcardiotomy ratings. Serum anticholinergic drug level is expressed as pmol/sample for a known amount of atropine. Displacement of [^{3}H]quinuclidinyl benzilate ([^{3}H]-QNB) is compared with an internal standard of atropine; it is then expressed as atropine equivalents.

ence was not statistically significant, but it did suggest that patients taking a greater number of drugs with mild anticholinergic properties may be more likely to become delirious.

Golinger et al. (1987) examined 25 patients admitted to a surgical intensive care unit over a 3-month period. Nine patients (36%) satisfied DSM-III criteria (American Psychiatric Association 1980) for delirium. Delirious patients had significantly higher plasma anticholinergic levels (4.67 ± 3.3 ng/ml) than did nondelirious patients (0.81 ± 1.0 ng/ml) ($t = 3.46$, $P = .007$).

3. Anticholinergic toxicity in the elderly.   Recent studies have focused on anticholinergic sensitivity and toxicity in the elderly. Miller et al. (1988) randomly assigned 18 psychiatrically healthy elderly patients to either a group receiving low dose of scopolamine as a presurgery medication or a control group receiving placebo. Pre- and postsurgical ratings included the Rey Auditory Verbal Learning Test, the Saskatoon Delirium Checklist, the MMSE score, and the Symbol-Digit Paired Associate Learning Test. Anticholinergic levels were determined by radioreceptor assay. Even though patients received very low doses of scopolamine (0.005 mg/kg), measurable serum anticholinergic levels were detected. The mean serum level was 9.1 ± 17.7 pmol/ml atropine equivalents. Anticholinergic drug levels were significantly associated with decreases in the Rey Auditory Verbal Learning Test when covariance-adjusted scores for scopolamine were compared with those of placebo ($t = 2.50$, df = 31, $P < .01$).

Rovner et al. (1988) investigated the effect of serum anticholinergic levels on cognition and self-care capacity in 22 demented nursing-home residents. Eleven patients satisfied DSM-III criteria for primary degenerative dementia, 9 had multi-infarct dementia, and 2 had other forms of dementia. The sample included 17 females and 5 men, with a mean age of 80.8 ± 9.6 years.

Patients identified as being at risk for developing anticholinergic toxicity were investigated. The entire sample received an average of 2.7 drugs per day. Clinical states were evaluated using the Psychogeriatric Dependency Rating Scales (PGDRS) (Wilkinson and Graham-White 1980). A wide range of anticholinergic drug levels was found (0.0–9.95 pmol/ml; median = 0.83 pmol/ml). Patients above and below the median anticholinergic level were then compared using PGDRS scores. Greater self-care impairment on the PGDRS was significantly correlated with

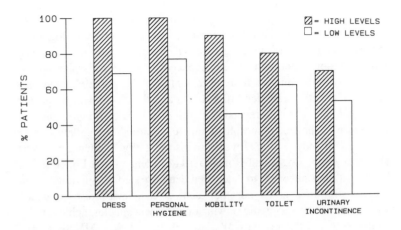

Figure 3–6. Comparison of specific activities-of-daily-living (ADL) dependencies and urinary incontinence in patients with high and low anticholinergic levels. The five items of the "self-care" subscale of the Psychogeriatric Dependency Rating Scales (PDGRS) (Wilkinson and Graham-White 1980) are presented. Patients are divided into two groups, those above (hatched bars) and those below (open bars) the median anticholinergic drug level (0.83 pmole/ml). Serum anticholinergic levels were significantly correlated with the total self-care scale (all five items combined) ($r = .42$, df = 20, $P < .025$).

higher serum anticholinergic drug level (see Figure 3-6). Self-care impairment reflected greater disability in dressing, personal hygiene, mobility, toileting, and urinary continence. The correlation between serum anticholinergic level and self-care score was statistically significant ($r = .42$, df = 20, $P < .025$).

4. Electroencephalography and anticholinergic delirium.

Because of the unavailability of the anticholinergic radioreceptor assay, we are currently investigating the use of a quantitative electroencephalogram (EEG), especially in patients who are both demented and delirious, as a possible way of measuring drug intoxication. An example of this approach (using the quantitative EEG) is illustrated in Figure 3-7. Demented patients evaluated in the DRC at the Johns Hopkins Hospital are being studied using both the EEG and serum anticholinergic drug levels.

The use of the quantitative EEG to identify delirious demented patients is based on the following argument. Electroencephalographic recordings are the only widely accepted diagnostic test for delirium. The most common abnormality of electroencephalographic morphology associated with delirium is the replacement of alpha (8–12 Hz) and beta (13–35 Hz) activity by delta (0.5–4 Hz) and theta (4–7 Hz) frequency activity. In patients with reversible delirium, the onset, progression, and resolution of the electroencephalographic abnormality parallel those of symptomatic indexes (e.g., severity of disorientation or attention deficit) (Brenner 1985; Engel and Romano 1944; Romano and Engel 1944). These parallels have not, to date, been demonstrated in individuals with a preexisting dementia syndrome, such as Alzheimer's disease, which itself results in characteristic slowing of electroencephalographic activity to the theta and delta ranges. We have obtained EEGs, MMSE scores, and anticholinergic drug levels from one such patient that demonstrate that this is indeed the case.

The following case example illustrates the use of the quantitative EEG to investigate drug toxicity in the elderly. A 69-year-old female patient with Alzheimer's disease became delirious after the administration of chloral hydrate for a sleep problem. Data were gathered during the delirium, and again 1 month later, after the medication had been stopped and the delirium had to a large extent remitted. Samples from the EEG for the delirious state and the remitted (i.e., partially recovered) state are presented in Figure 3-7. At the time of the recording in the delirious state, the patient's MMSE score was 15, and her serum anticholinergic level was 2.47 ng/ml.

Electroencephalographic tracings are comprised primarily of low-frequency, high-amplitude activity—particularly in frontal areas (see Figure 3-7, left). Power spectral analysis revealed that 75%–80% of EEG power fell within the delta and theta frequency ranges. On recovery, the patient's MMSE score increased by 7 points to 22, the serum anticholinergic level was 0.0, and the amount of slow EEG activity decreased (Figure 3-7, right).

Comparing this record to that obtained during the delirious state, EEG power in the theta band decreased 10%, theta frequency increased from 4 Hz to 7 Hz, and beta-band power increased by 8.6% with the resolution of delirium. Theta activity remained quite prominent in the EEG record, which is a characteristic of electroencephalographic activity in patients with Alzheimer's disease. These data indicate that quantita-

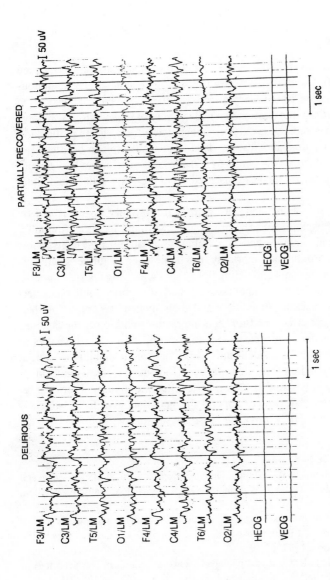

Figure 3–7. Electroencephalographic activity recorded from a 69-year-old female patient with Alzheimer's disease and concurrent drug-induced delirium (left) while the patient was delirious, as determined by delta and slow (4-Hz) theta activity; and (right) upon resolution of the delirium, when the theta frequency was increased (7 Hz) and the delta activity was reduced.

tive analysis of electroencephalographic activity yields important information related to the course and severity of delirium in patients with dementia.

Summary

We now have over 2,300 years experience with anticholinergic-induced delirium. The studies reviewed in this chapter indicate the ubiquitous nature of this syndrome. They underscore the importance of considering therapeutic drug intoxication in a wide variety of patient groups. In most of the studies reviewed, elderly patients were found to be particularly vulnerable to drug intoxication. This is generally felt to be related to age-related declines in cholinergic neurotransmission and to the increased number of medications used by the elderly (Blass and Plum 1982).

Delirium is associated with increased morbidity (as measured by prolonged hospital stay [Thomas et al. 1988]) and increased mortality (Gottleib et al., unpublished data; Rabins and Folstein 1982). Given this increased morbidity and mortality, the importance of further characterization of the problem and defining ways of identifying the syndrome, as well as its risk factors, cannot be overstated. It is important to characterize commonly used compounds and their metabolites, both for their anticholinergic effects and for their interactions with other medications at the acetylcholine receptors. One major limitation of most studies of anticholinergic-induced delirium is the lack of availability of serum anticholinergic drug levels. Our recent efforts have focused on developing alternative ways of assessing anticholinergic toxicity. From the results in Figure 3-7, we are hopeful that a quantitative EEG, which is widely available, may provide at least one satisfactory option.

References

American Psychiatric Association: Diagnostic and Statistical Manual of Mental Disorders, 3rd Edition. Washington, DC, American Psychiatric Association, 1980

American Psychiatric Association: Diagnostic and Statistical Manual of Mental Disorders, 3rd Edition, Revised. Washington, DC, American Psychiatric Association, 1987

Blass J, Plum F: Metabolic encephalopathies in older adults, in The Neurology of Aging. Edited by Plum F. New York, FA Davis, 1982, pp 189–219

Blazer DG, Federspiel CF, Ray WA, et al: The risk of anticholinergic toxicity in the elderly: a study of prescribing practices in two populations. Journal of Geriatrics 38:31–35, 1983

Brenner RP: The electroencephalogram in altered states of consciousness. Neurol Clin 3:615–631, 1985

Cahn L, Diesfeldt H: The use of neuroleptics in the treatment of dementia in old age. Psychiatr Neurol Neurochir (Amst) 76:411–420, 1973

DiMascio A, Bernardo DL, Greenblatt DJ, et al: A controlled trial of amantadine in drug-induced extrapyramidal disorders. Arch Gen Psychiatry 33:599–602, 1976

Engel GL, Romano J: Delirium, II: reversibility of the electroencephalogram with experimental procedures. Archives of Neurology and Psychiatry 51:378–392, 1944

Folstein MF, Folstein SE, McHugh PR: "Mini-Mental State": a practical method for grading the cognitive state of patients for the clinician. J Psychiatr Res 12:189–198, 1975

Golinger RC, Peet T, Tune LE: Association of elevated plasma anticholinergic activity with delirium in surgical patients. Am J Psychiatry 144:1218–1220, 1987

Gotestam K, Ljunghall S, Olsson B: A double-blind comparison of the effects of haloperidol and cis(z)-clopenthixol in senile dementia. Acta Psychiatr Scand Suppl 294:46–51, 1981

Lipowski ZJ: Delirium: Acute Brain Failure in Man, 2nd Edition. Springfield, IL, Charles C Thomas, 1990

McKhann GM, Drachman D, Folstein M, et al: Clinical diagnosis of Alzheimer's disease: report of the NINCDS/ADRDA Workgroup under the auspices of the Department of Health and Human Services Task Force on Alzheimer's Disease. Neurology 34:939–944, 1984

Miller PS, Richardson JS, Jyu CA, et al: Association of low serum anticholinergic levels and cognitive impairment in elderly presurgical patients. Am J Psychiatry 145:342–345, 1988

Rabins PV, Folstein MF: Delirium and dementia: diagnostic criteria and fatality rates. Br J Psychiatry 140:149–153, 1982

Steele C, Lucas MJ, Tune L: Haloperidol versus thioridazine in the treatment of behavioral symptoms in senile dementia of the Alzheimer's type: preliminary findings. J Clin Psychiatry 47(6):310–312, 1986

Summers WR: A clinical method of estimating risk of drug-induced delirium. Life Sci 22:1511–1516, 1978

Thomas RI, Cameron DJ, Fahs M: A prospective study of delirium and prolonged hospital stay: exploratory study. Arch Gen Psychiatry 45:937–940, 1988

Tune LE, Coyle JT: Acute extrapyramidal side effects: serum levels of neuroleptics and anticholinergics. Psychopharmacology (Berlin) 95:9–15, 1981

Tune L, Holland A, Folstein M, et al: Association of post-operative delirium with raised level anticholinergic drugs. Lancet 2:650–652, 1981

Tune L, Steele C, Cooper T: Neuroleptic drugs in the management of behavioral symptoms of Alzheimer's disease. Psychiatr Clin North Am 14:353–373, 1991

Wilkinson IM, Graham-White J: Psychogeriatric dependency rating scales (PGDRS): a method of assessment for use by nurses. Br J Psychiatry 137:558–565, 1980

Chapter 4

Neuroleptic Malignant Syndrome in the Elderly

Gerard Addonizio, M.D.

Neuroleptic malignant syndrome (NMS) is a potentially lethal disorder associated with the use of neuroleptic medication. The syndrome is characterized by extrapyramidal symptoms and hyperthermia and is often associated with agitation, confusion, diaphoresis, leukocytosis, elevated creatine phosphokinase (CPK) levels, autonomic instability, and incontinence (Addonizio et al. 1987). The frequency of NMS in patients on neuroleptics has been estimated to be between 0.07% and 1.4% (Addonizio and Susman 1991). Neuroleptic malignant syndrome has been reported to occur in young men more frequently than young women. The disorder has been seen in patients from childhood to the geriatric population.

Although NMS was considered largely a problem in young adults, it has now become clear that patients of all ages are affected. The psychiatric diagnosis in most reported cases has been either schizophrenia or bipolar disorder. Patients with organic brain disease are probably more sensitive to the development of NMS (Addonizio et al. 1987). In most cases, high-potency neuroleptics such as haloperidol have been implicated, but many cases have been reported in which low-potency neuroleptics such as chlorpromazine were used. Rapid increases in neuroleptic dose, as well as parenteral administration of a neuroleptic, appear to enhance the possibility of development of NMS (Keck et al. 1989). Simultaneous use of lithium may also be a risk factor. There have been a number of reports of patients with Parkinson's disease developing a syndrome identical to NMS when antiparkinsonian medication was abruptly withdrawn even though these patients had not received a neuroleptic (Friedman et al. 1985). Therefore, the syndrome of NMS may be caused by a sudden decrease in dopaminergic function through dopamine-receptor blockade or through a sudden loss of a needed dopaminergic agent.

Neuroleptic Malignant Syndrome: An Overview

Clinical Signs and Laboratory Findings

In NMS, elevated temperature ranges from minor elevations to marked hyperthermic states. Extrapyramidal symptoms include rigidity, tremors, and dystonias. These symptoms usually appear before or concomitant with the development of elevated temperature, suggesting that at least part of the hyperthermia is caused by muscle-generated heat. Tachycardia is commonly found, and blood pressure is often elevated, although both diastolic and systolic pressures can become labile. Confusion is commonly reported, sometimes reaching severe delirium. Agitation further complicates the clinical picture. Incontinence is occasionally described. Because of their agitated, confused states, patients with NMS often have poor oral intake and subsequently become quite dehydrated. Dehydration is often mentioned as a risk factor for NMS and may also be a consequence of the illness.

Elevated levels of CPK are frequently seen but may also be caused by intramuscular injections, muscle trauma, and use of restraints. Increased CPK has also been correlated to the acutely psychotic state (Meltzer et al. 1980). In NMS, elevations may be minimal, but they may also reach extremely high levels, sometimes into the thousands. High levels of CPK may be the harbinger of severe rhabdomyolysis and myoglobinuric renal failure. Leukocytosis is commonly observed with a range of 10,000–40,000/mm^3. Analysis of cerebrospinal fluid is usually normal, and computed tomography (CT) scans only show incidental findings. Also, electroencephalograms may exhibit nonspecific slowing.

Case example.   Mr. A., a 75-year-old man with a history of bipolar disorder, was admitted to an inpatient psychiatric unit in a manic state after he had stopped taking lithium. He was agitated and belligerent and exhibited flight of ideas, grandiose delusions, a markedly labile affect, and an elevated mood. He was placed on haloperidol, 8 mg/day, and benztropine mesylate (Cogentin), 0.5 mg twice daily. Within 48 hours he became tremulous, rigid, diaphoretic, and confused. He developed tachycardia and labile blood pressure, and his temperature rose to 103°F. His white blood cell (WBC) count rose to 14,000/mm^3, and his CPK was measured at 900 IU/liter. A thorough medical workup, including blood cultures, analysis of cerebrospinal fluid, and CT scan, was unremarkable and no focus of infection was discovered. As NMS was diagnosed, haloperidol was immediately discontinued, and supportive medical care, including adequate hydration, was instituted. Over the next several days all autonomic, extrapyramidal, and laboratory abnormalities gradually normalized, and the patient reached his baseline pretreated state within 10 days following discontinuation of haloperidol.

Clinical Course and Complications

Neuroleptic malignant syndrome may occur at any time during neuroleptic treatment but most commonly occurs during the first 2 weeks of receiving neuroleptic medication (Addonizio et al. 1987). The syndrome may occur in a full-blown form over the course of several hours or may gradually progress in a more insidious fashion over the course of several days. After NMS has developed, discontinuing neuroleptics usually leads to resolution of the disorder within a mean duration of 2 weeks for nondepot medication and 1 month for depot preparations. Medical complications that can affect the clinical course include pneumonia, renal failure, cardiac arrest, seizures, sepsis, and pulmonary embolism. Mortality rates based on a series of published cases range from 10% to 20% (Addonizio et al. 1987), but these fatality rates may largely reflect reporting biases of the published cases.

Differential Diagnosis

Distinguishing between NMS and lethal catatonia is probably the most difficult task in the differential diagnosis of NMS. The two disorders can present in virtually indistinguishable ways (Mann et al. 1986). Making the correct diagnosis is crucial, as continuing neuroleptics in a patient with NMS may have lethal consequences.

Malignant hyperthermia also has similar symptoms, but making the diagnosis of malignant hyperthermia should be relatively easy, because this disorder occurs with the administration of halogenated inhalational anesthetics and the depolarizing muscle relaxant succinylcholine (Nelson and Flewellen 1983). Malignant hyperthermia is more fulminant in onset and carries a very high mortality rate. Heat stroke, sometimes seen in patients on neuroleptics, can usually be differentiated from NMS by the absence of diaphoresis and rigidity.

Other disorders that may mimic NMS include severe dystonia, central nervous system infection, akinetic mutism, "locked-in syndrome," tetany, thyrotoxicosis, pheochromocytoma, intermittent acute porphyria, and tetanus. Pharmacologic agents that may be associated with NMS-like syndromes include sudden withdrawal of antiparkinsonian medication in a patient with Parkinson's disease, monoamine oxidase inhibitors, combinations of monoamine oxidase inhibitors and other antidepressants, lithium toxicity, anticholinergic delirium, amphetamines, fenfluramine, cocaine, phencyclidine (PCP), and strychnine. In most cases, a careful history and physical exam will help to distinguish these disorders from NMS.

Treatment and Aftercare

Immediate discontinuation of neuroleptic medications and supportive medical treatment (e.g., rehydration and cooling) are the mainstay of management of NMS. In most patients this type of treatment will be sufficient. With other patients who develop a more severe form of NMS, it may be necessary to attempt treatment with other pharmacological agents. Bromocriptine, a dopamine agonist, has been used with some success (Figa-Talamanca et al. 1985). Amantadine, an indirect dopamine agonist, has also been efficacious in some cases (Gangadhar et al. 1984). Based on its therapeutic usefulness in treating malignant hyperthermia, some clinicians have used the muscle relaxant dantrolene (Greenberg and Gujavarty 1985). Although all of these medicines have been used with some success, the degree of their efficacy remains undetermined, because most of the data are derived from case reports. Because NMS is usually a self-limited disorder (Addonizio et al. 1986), it is unclear how many of the cases would have resolved without resorting to pharmacological interventions.

Case example.   Mrs. B., a 76-year-old woman with a primary degenerative dementia, was admitted to an inpatient psychiatric unit in a severely agitated state. On admission she exhibited paranoid delusions and was extremely belligerent with staff. She was placed on haloperidol, 1 mg tid. Within 72 hours she became rigid, tremulous, confused, incontinent, and tachycardic, with an elevation in both systolic and diastolic blood pressure. Her temperature rose to 102.8°F, and her WBC count and CPK levels were minimally elevated. A thorough medical workup revealed no source of infection. A CT scan of the head was normal except for moderate atrophy and ventricular dilatation. The diagnosis of NMS was made and haloperidol was discontinued. Two days later, symptoms of NMS continued unabated. Treatment with bromocriptine, 2.5 mg tid, was instituted, and within 48 hours there was an improvement in extrapyramidal and autonomic disturbances. Within 8 days the patient was no longer rigid or tremulous, and her temperature, blood pressure, and pulse normalized.

Patients who have had NMS often have recurrences when neuroleptic medications are reintroduced (Susman and Addonizio 1988). Currently, the safest strategy appears to be restarting treatment with low doses of low-potency neuroleptics after a minimum of 2 weeks following resolution of symptoms of NMS. Concomitantly these patients must be followed closely for any signs of recurrence. For patients who cannot tolerate neuroleptics, other treatments such as electroconvulsive therapy may be helpful (Addonizio and Susman 1987). In the post-NMS period, lithium may be considered, but this agent has been reported to reinduce NMS (Susman and Addonizio 1987).

Neuroleptic Malignant Syndrome in the Elderly

For a period of time NMS was thought to occur primarily in young individuals (Caroff 1980). A reading of the literature led one to believe that the elderly were relatively immune. More recently it has become clear that this notion is untrue (Addonizio 1987). In one review of 115 cases of NMS, Addonizio et al. reported that the mean age was 40 years (range 12–71 years), with 51% of the cases under 40 years of age (Addonizio and Susman 1987). A recently updated review of 288 NMS cases in the literature showed that 246 cases were under 60 years of age while 42 (15%) cases were 60 years old or above (Addonizio and Susman 1991). Dementia was the diagnosis in 8 cases, while in 9 cases there was a diagnosis of Parkinson's disease. Five of the patients with Parkinson's disease developed symptoms of NMS on no neuroleptic when antiparkinsonian medication was withdrawn. Of the 42 cases of NMS, the fatality rate was 29% (25% if patients with Parkinson's disease on no neuroleptic are excluded). Although fatality rates cannot be determined on the basis of case reports, it is important to note that this figure is higher than the usually quoted 10%–20% fatality rate for all patients based on similar reviews of the literature.

There are a number of reasons why older patients may actually be at risk for developing NMS (Addonizio and Susman 1991). High-potency neuroleptic medications (e.g., haloperidol) are most commonly used in the elderly because of their relative lack of cardiovascular effects. On the other hand, high-potency neuroleptics are implicated more frequently in cases of NMS. Organic brain disease, a potential risk factor for NMS, is much more common in the elderly as a result of Alzheimer's disease and cerebral infarcts. Dehydration, another factor potentiating the development of NMS, is also commonly found in elderly patients whose oral intake has markedly diminished.

Another risk factor for this age group is a greater difficulty in maintaining thermeostasis (Collins 1985). Structural and functional changes in the nervous system and in decreased blood supply to central and peripheral effector systems impair the efficiency of thermoregulatory processes. These changes also make it more difficult to handle external heat loads. Consequently, high ambient temperature as well as impaired thermoregulatory processes could increase the risk of NMS in the older individual. In addition, the ability to decrease body temperature is further impaired, because the elderly have been shown to have a reduced sweating response following thermal and neurochemical stimulation compared with that of young adults (Collins 1985). Older individuals are also at greater risk for developing the medical complications of NMS. Pneumonia, pulmonary embolism, renal failure, and cardiorespiratory arrest are all more likely to have fatal consequences in the elderly population.

Making the diagnosis of NMS in the older patient may be more difficult than in the younger patient. Based on physiological changes that occur with aging, symptoms of NMS may be obscured or incorrectly interpreted (Addonizio and Susman 1991). Tremors and rigidity are commonly found in patients with degenerative dementia. Similarly, confusion is often seen in patients with dementia. Incontinence is seen much more frequently in elderly patients and consequently does not arouse the same type of concern it would in a young patient. Clearly, most patients with any of these symptoms do not necessarily have NMS, but sudden onset of these symptoms should alert the clinician to the potential development of NMS. Impaired thermoregulatory responses may impair the development of high temperatures, an essential feature of NMS that is often the most critical warning sign signaling the disorder.

Lability of blood pressure, another frequent feature of NMS, is all too common a finding in elderly patients on psychotropic medication. Sudden elevations of blood pressure should be seen as a potential warning sign and not immediately labeled as an age-related change in systolic pressure. Frail elderly patients often have poor nutritional intake and decreased muscle mass, making it difficult to develop a significant leukocytosis or increase in CPK.

Over the past several years it has become clear that NMS is not only a disorder of young adults but also a disorder that may affect older patients, sometimes in a devastating way. Furthermore, the elderly may be at risk for the development of NMS and will respond more adversely to medical complications. Because the presentation of NMS may be different in older individuals because of age-related physiological changes, it is important for clinicians treating patients in this age group to be keenly aware of signs and symptoms that may signal the development of this potentially lethal disorder.

References

Addonizio G: Neuroleptic malignant syndrome in elderly patients. J Am Geriatr Soc 35:1011–1012, 1987

Addonizio G, Susman VL: ECT as a treatment alternative for patients with symptoms of neuroleptic malignant syndrome. J Clin Psychiatry 48(3):102–105, 1987

Addonizio G, Susman VL: Neuroleptic Malignant Syndrome: A Clinical Approach. St. Louis, MO, Mosby–Year Book, 1991

Addonizio G, Susman VL, Roth SD: Symptoms of neuroleptic malignant syndrome in 82 consecutive inpatients. Am J Psychiatry 143:1587–1590, 1986

Addonizio G, Susman VL, Roth SD: Neuroleptic malignant syndrome: review and analysis of 115 cases. Biol Psychiatry 22:1004–1020, 1987

Caroff SN: The neuroleptic malignant syndrome. J Clin Psychiatry 41:79–83, 1980

Collins KJ: Disorders of homeostasis, in Practical Geriatric Medicine. Edited by Exton-Smith AN, Weksler ME. Edinburgh, Churchill Livingstone, 1985, pp 74–83

Figa-Talamanca L, Gualandi C, DiMeo L, et al: Hyperthermia after discontinuance of levodopa and bromocriptine therapy: impaired dopamine receptors a possible cause. Neurology 35:258–261, 1985

Friedman JH, Feinberg SS, Feldman RG: A neuroleptic malignant-like syndrome due to levodopa therapy withdrawal. JAMA 254:2792–2795, 1985

Gangadhar BN, Desai NG, Channabasavanna SM: Amantadine in the neuroleptic malignant syndrome (letter). J Clin Psychiatry 45:526, 1984

Greenberg LB, Gujavarty K: The neuroleptic malignant syndrome: review and report of three cases. Compr Psychiatry 26:63–70, 1985

Keck PE Jr, Pope HG Jr, Cohen BM, et al: Risk factors for neuroleptic malignant syndrome: a case-control study. Arch Gen Psychiatry 46:914–918, 1989

Mann SC, Caroff SN, Bleier HR, et al: Lethal catatonia. Am J Psychiatry 143:1374–1381, 1986

Meltzer HY, Ross-Stanton J, Schlessinger S: Mean serum creatine kinase activity in patients with functional psychoses. Arch Gen Psychiatry 37:650–655, 1980

Nelson TE, Flewellen EH: Current concepts: the malignant hyperthermia syndrome. N Engl J Med 309:416–418, 1983

Susman VL, Addonizio G: Reinduction of neuroleptic malignant syndrome by lithium. J Clin Psychopharmacol 7:339–341, 1987

Susman VL, Addonizio G: Recurrence of neuroleptic malignant syndrome. J Nerv Ment Dis 176:234–241, 1988

Chapter 5

Problems Associated With Long-Term Benzodiazepine Use in the Elderly

Javaid I. Sheikh, M.D.

Since their introduction in the early 1960s, benzodiazepines have become the most prescribed of all psychotropic medications for more than two decades (Grantham 1987; Sussman and Chou 1988). Statistics compiled by the National Institute on Drug Abuse (1986) indicate that 6 of the top 25 prescribed drugs are benzodiazepines. A survey conducted in August 1987 (Louis Harris and Associates 1987) found that 11% of the population had received a prescription for a sedative or tranquilizer in the past 12 months. It was also found that these prescriptions were almost exclusively for benzodiazepines, and of those individuals currently taking benzodiazepines, 31% had been using them for a year or more. Similar patterns are described for England. Grantham (1987) notes that 10% of adult males and 20% of adult females in England were taking a benzodiazepine at some point during the course of a year in the 1970s and 1980s. Such popularity of benzodiazepines can be ascribed partly to the multiple usages of these medications, including their use as sedative-hypnotics, anxiolytics, muscle relaxants, anticonvulsants, and anesthetics. In comparison with their predecessors, such as alcohol, barbiturates, and propanediols (e.g., meprobamate), benzodiazepines are safer and at least as effective.

Various reports in the literature indicating that abuse and dependence quite frequently can be associated with long-term benzodiazepine use have stirred debates about the advantages and disadvantages of benzodiazepines (Burch 1990; Grantham 1987; Uhlenhuth et al. 1988; Woods et al. 1988). Abuse and dependence issues are particularly relevant to the elderly, because there is an indication that long-term benzodiazepine use is particularly common in this age group (Mellinger et al. 1984). It also appears that the elderly may be particularly vulnerable to the side effects of benzodiazepines, such as drowsiness, cognitive suppression, and psychomotor impairment (Boston Collaborative Drug Surveillance Program 1973; Kanto et al. 1981; Pomara et al. 1991). In this chapter I will review findings from the literature on patterns of usage of benzodiazepines in the elderly, critically examine and describe the clinical implications of problems associated with long-term usage, suggest ways to curtail inappropriate use of these medications, and suggest alternative interventions for coping with anxiety and insomnia, for which those medications are prescribed most commonly in the elderly.

Patterns of Usage of Benzodiazepines

Various estimates suggest that older adults aged 65 and above, comprising approximately 12% of the population, use 25%–40% of the prescription drugs, most commonly cardiovascular drugs, hypnotics, anxiolytics, and analgesics (Moran et al. 1988; Rowe and Besdine 1982; Stephens et al. 1982). Of hypnotics and anxiolytics, benzodiazepines are the most commonly prescribed medications, both for the general population and for the elderly (Balter et al. 1984; Moran et al. 1988). As expected, surveys suggest that the elderly get prescriptions of benzodiazepines in disproportionately high numbers compared with their percentage in the general population. For example, the National Disease and Therapeutic Index (NDTI) (1986) has established that 40% of prescriptions for benzodiazepine hypnotics and 26% of prescriptions for benzodiazepine anxiolytics are given to the elderly. In addition, it appears that as many as one-third of elderly patients hospitalized for a medical illness receive a benzodiazepine (Shaw and Opit 1976).

In a national survey conducted in the United States in 1979 with a cross-sectional sample of 3,161 noninstitutionalized adults ranging in age from 18 to 79, 11.1% of the people reported taking a prescribed anxiolytic one or more times in the last 12 months (Mellinger et al. 1984). Two-thirds of these people described using an anxiolytic occasionally or on a daily basis for less than a month, whereas 15% described a daily intake of anxiolytics for more than 12 months. Fully 71% of the long-term users were ages 50 and above, and one-third were above 65 years of age. In addition, 61% were females. Finally, significantly more long-term users than nonusers scored high on a standard scale of psychological distress, and 75% of long-term users reported two or more health problems, particularly cardiovascular or musculoskeletal disorders.

Similar findings have been reported from England in a survey of long-term usage of benzodiazepines (Morgan et al. 1988). In a nationally representative sample of 1,020 community-dwelling older adults aged 65 and over, over 16% of the sample reported using hypnotic drugs (mostly benzodiazepines) sometimes. A significant majority of these users (71%) reported hypnotic use for more than 1 year, and a full 25% reported such use for more than 10 years. Similar to the findings of Mellinger et al. (1984) in the United States, female sex and increasing age seemed to correlate with increasing use. Higher rates for hypnotic intake (15%–50%) in "old people's homes" (i.e., nursing homes) have also been reported by Oswald (1984). Finally, Williamson and Chopin (1980) report that in England up to 22% of the elderly with a physical illness receive a benzodiazepine on an ongoing basis. Thus, it appears that long-term usage of benzodiazepines as sedative-hypnotics and/or anxiolytics is rather widespread in the elderly.

Drug Disposition Problems

In order to fully comprehend the scope of problems associated with long-term benzodiazepine use in the elderly, it will be helpful to review some physiological changes occurring as part of normal aging. These changes in absorption, distribution, protein binding, metabolism, and excretion of drugs can lead to excessive accumulation of benzodiazepines in the body tissues of the elderly, predisposing these individuals to undesirable side effects.

Briefly, drug absorption may be altered on account of decreases in splanchnic blood flow, increases in gastric pH, and changes in active and passive transport (Omslander 1981). Concomitant use of antacids, not uncommon in the elderly, can impede absorption of benzodiazepines. An increase in proportion of body fat with aging affects distribution of lipophilic compounds such as benzodiazepines into tissues and across the blood-brain barrier. Within benzodiazepines, lipid solubility varies greatly, and a strongly lipophilic drug like diazepam may lead to a much higher accumulation in tissues compared with a less lipophilic drug like lorazepam (Moran et al. 1988). A reduction in serum albumin may mean more free drug in plasma, especially if there is dietary insufficiency or chronic illness, so there is a greater chance of undesirable side effects

(Greenblatt et al. 1989). A decrease in hepatic metabolism may further increase levels of unmetabolized drug, especially longer-acting benzodiazepines that depend on oxidation (Lavizzo-Mourey 1989). Finally, a gradual decrease in glomerular filtration rate (GFR) and renal blood flow to 50% in the elderly by the age of 70 (as compared with that of a 40-year-old) means slower clearance of drugs (Papper 1978).

Clinical Usage of Benzodiazepines

As noted previously, benzodiazepines are most frequently used as sedative-hypnotics and anxiolytics, and less frequently for other medical uses such as anticonvulsants, muscle relaxants, and anesthetics (Sussman 1985). As anxiolytics, they have been the mainstay of treatment for anxiety disorders for more than two decades, and there is sufficient evidence that benzodiazepines are quite effective in anxious older people as well (Hershey and Kim 1988; Sheikh 1991). As hypnotics, benzodiazepines are again the most frequently prescribed compounds (Moran et al. 1988). As noted earlier, the elderly are prescribed benzodiazepines at a rate disproportionately high to their percentage in the population. This high rate is somewhat understandable, because both anxiety and insomnia appear to be very common in this age group (Blazer et al. 1991; Gottlieb 1990; Sheikh 1991). Table 5-1 lists commonly used anxiolytic and hypnotic benzodiazepines, along with relevant information about their half-lives and the daily doses recommended for the elderly.

Short-Acting Versus Long-Acting Benzodiazepines

It seems logical for geriatricians to look in a specific class of compounds for drugs that are not significantly affected much in terms of metabolism by the physiological changes associated with aging. Of the benzodiazepines, it appears that lorazepam, oxazepam, and temazepam are inactivated by direct conjugation in the liver, a mechanism that does not seem to be affected by aging (Greenblatt et al. 1989). In addition, these drugs are relatively less lipophilic and are thus less prone to accumulate in fatty tissues of the elderly compared with a more lipophilic drug such as diazepam (Moran et al. 1988). Because of these factors, the half-lives of

Table 5–1. Commonly used benzodiazepines

Drug	Half-life (hours)	Active metabolites	Average daily dose (mg) Adult	Elderly
Anxiolytics				
Alprazolam	12–15	Yes	0.25–2.0	0.125–1
Chlordiazepoxide	7–28	Yes	25–100	5–50
Clonazepam	18–56	Yes	1–8	0.5–4
Clorazepate	30–200	Yes	15–60	7.5–30
Diazepam	20–60	Yes	5–30	2–15
Lorazepam	10–20	None	1–6	0.5–3
Halazepam	15–50	Yes	20–160	20–80
Oxazepam	5–15	None	15–9	10–45
Prazepam	25–200	Yes	20–60	10–20
Hypnotics				
Flurazepam	50–200	Yes	30	15
Temazepam	8–10	None	30	15
Triazolam	2.5	Yes	0.25–0.50	0.125–0.25

these benzodiazepines are relatively short (see Table 5-1) in both the young and the old. Most other benzodiazepines tend to be metabolized via oxidative pathways into active metabolites that tend to linger on in the elderly for long periods of time. For example, flurazepam, a commonly used hypnotic, is metabolized through oxidation to desalkylflurazepam, an active metabolite with a half-life of approximately 65 hours in the young and up to 100 to 200 hours in the elderly (Greenblatt et al. 1981).

Similar findings have been described for other long-acting benzodiazepines such as diazepam, clorazepate, and prazepam (Cutler and Narang 1984). For example, Rosenbaum (1979) documents that the half-life of diazepam's metabolites increases from 20 hours in a 20-year-old to 90 hours in an 80-year-old. Alprazolam is an intermediate-acting drug whose mean half-life in one study was shown to increase from 11 hours in young people to 19 hours in elderly men, but was not shown to increase at the same rate in elderly women (Greenblatt et al. 1983). However, Kroboth et al. (1990) reported mean half-lives of alprazolam in excess of 21 hours in *both* elderly men and elderly women and reduced oral clearance values in the elderly (to 55%–82% of those in young adults). These authors also reported that tolerance to the sedative effects of alprazolam develops more slowly in the elderly, suggesting less adaptive receptor mechanisms.

Clinical implications of this review are that short-acting benzodiazepines such as oxazepam, lorazepam, and temazepam are clearly preferable in the elderly, especially because they do not have active metabolites. Long-acting benzodiazepines such as diazepam, clorazepate, and flurazepam appear to be less desirable in general.

Potential Complications of Long-Term Benzodiazepine Use

Various problems can occur with long-term benzodiazepine use in the elderly (see Table 5-2). A brief review of the literature documenting the nature and extent of these complications is presented below.

Daytime Sedation

Daytime sedation is a commonly observed problem in clinical situations, although it is often ignored. Surveys of inpatients treated with benzodiazepines suggest that the elderly may show more drowsiness, fatigue, and ataxia compared with younger patients (Boston Collaborative Drug Surveillance Program 1973; Greenblatt and Allen 1978). The elderly also self-report more sedation compared with younger people after treatment with benzodiazepines (Kanto et al. 1981). Next-day sedation and cognitive impairment have also been reported in the elderly after one night, five nights, and eight nights of treatment with nitrazepam, a commonly used

Table 5–2.   Potential complications of long-term benzodiazepine use in the elderly

Excessive daytime drowsiness
Cognitive impairment and confusion
Psychomotor impairment and a risk of falls
Paradoxical reactions
Depression
Intoxication, even on therapeutic dosages
Amnestic syndromes
Respiratory problems
Abuse and dependence
Breakthrough withdrawal reactions

hypnotic (Kanto et al. 1981; Murphy et al. 1982). It also appears that the elderly show sedation at substantially lower concentrations of benzodiazepines than do younger people (Reidenberg et al. 1978). Given the longer elimination periods for benzodiazepines in the elderly, their lipophilic nature, and their consequent accumulation over a period of time, and possibly the increased sensitivity of the elderly to their side effects (Lavizzo-Mourey 1989), long-term use of hypnotics, especially the long-acting ones, does not seem to be appropriate in this population. It is worth noting that the Committee on Safety of Medicines (1988) in the United Kingdom strongly advises against use of benzodiazepine hypnotics for longer than 4 weeks in all age groups.

Cognitive Impairment

Studies have documented cognitive impairment from single and multiple doses of benzodiazepines as manifested by problems in arousal, attention, acquisition of new information, and a decline in motor performance in both young and elderly subjects (Pomara et al. 1990; Taylor and Tinklenberg 1987). In a placebo-controlled study comparing 45 normal young subjects (age range 19–35) with 45 normal elderly subjects (age range 60–79 years), Pomara et al. (1990) documented acute and significant cognitive impairment in memory, attention, and reaction time in both the young and the old subjects, with a trend for greater impairment in the elderly, after ingestion of 10 mg diazepam. These authors also reported that older, but not younger, patients showed deficits in response to 2.5 mg of diazepam. In addition, 10 mg of diazepam given nightly for 1 and 3 weeks produced comparable next-day cognitive deficits between groups. This study also suggested only partial tolerance in both age groups to acute effects of diazepam after 3 weeks of treatment.

These findings indicate that the elderly may be vulnerable to undesirable side effects at doses of benzodiazepines considered "safe" and "low" for younger people. A recent report also suggests that there is some decline in the adaptive capacity of the elderly to adjust to the adverse effects of benzodiazepines over a period of time (Nikaido et al. 1990).

In a population in which many members may already be experiencing cognitive decline associated with age (Craik 1977), additional cognitive suppression as a result of benzodiazepine use may produce serious cognitive impairment and dysfunction. It can also lead to unnecessary panic on the part of spouses or other family members who might mistake it for a dementing process.

Psychomotor Impairment

Investigators have reported psychomotor impairment in long-term benzodiazepine users as evidenced by deficits in choice reaction time, critical fusion flicker thresholds, digit symbol substitution, and symbol copying (Hindmarch and Clyde 1980; Petursson et al. 1983). Some inferential evidence of such impairment is also provided by a survey suggesting that the chances of getting into a serious automobile accident are five times greater for benzodiazepine users as compared with nonusers (Skegg et al. 1979). Other studies also suggest that the probability of getting into a fatal collision is higher in benzodiazepine users compared with the risk for users of alcohol, antihistamines, or cannabinoids (Warren 1981). Similar results have been reported in Norway (Bo et al. 1975). One has to interpret such large-scale surveys with caution because of a lack of control for many important variables, including the presence of psychopathology, past history of accidents, and the duration and frequency of benzodiazepine use. Such findings do indicate, however, a reason for caution in prescribing such medications to a population whose coordination may not be as good to begin with as younger persons'.

Another related issue is the risk of falls associated with long-term benzodiazepine use. Sorock and Shimkin (1988) reported in a prospective study of 169 ambulatory tenants of six senior citizen buildings in New Jersey that continuous use of benzodiazepines is associated with a higher risk of falling compared with nonuse or prn use. Similar results have also been reported for nursing home residents who are sedative users of mostly long-acting benzodiazepines, with the relative risk of falling ranging from 1.8 to 3.1 compared with nonusers of sedatives (Granek et al. 1987; Sobel and McCart 1983).

Taking this line of reasoning further, Ray and associates (1987) studied an elderly sample of Medicaid enrollees in Michigan and found a relative risk of hip fracture of 1.8 in subjects using long-half-life benzodiazepines compared with the nonusers. They did not find any increased risk among current users of short-half-life hypnotics and anxiolytics (mostly nonbenzodiazepines). The same group of investigators later reported a retrospective case-control study in a large sample of elderly comparing the risk of hip fracture in users of long-half-life (24 hours or more) benzodiazepines versus short-half-life (less than 24 hours) benzodiazepines (Ray et al. 1989). The risk for hip fracture relative to the nonusers was 1.7 for current users of long-half-life benzodiazepines compared with 1.1 for current users of short-half-life benzodiazepines. These findings remained consistent when subjects were controlled for age, sex, nursing home residence, and history of hospitalization. Such findings suggest that clinicians should exercise caution in prescribing any long-acting benzodiazepines in the elderly.

Psychiatric Complications

Benzodiazepines are central nervous system depressants and thus may cause or exacerbate existing depression. Lydiard et al. (1987) reported findings from a study in which one-third of panic disorder patients developed symptoms of major depression after a few weeks of treatment with alprazolam. In addition, it appears that long-term use of these medications may be associated with a blunting of emotional response (Lader and Petursson 1981). According to Grantham (1987), there might be a rebound effect when these medications are discontinued, leading to explosive expression of feelings suppressed for a long period of time. In clinical situations, such "emotional incontinence" may lead to a long and fruitless search for an underlying neurological condition in an elderly patient unless a careful history of benzodiazepine use is taken.

Paradoxical Reactions

There are rare cases of paradoxical reactions secondary to benzodiazepine use. Such reactions usually consist of aggressive behavior (Lader and Petursson 1981). There are also reports of antisocial acts such as shoplifting being associated with long-term benzodiazepine use (Ashton 1986). In addition, there are reports of other paradoxical reactions to benzodiazepines, including insomnia and nightmares, especially with triazolam (Moran et al. 1988). Geriatricians need to be aware of such infrequent but potentially cumbersome occurrences.

Drug Interactions

Benzodiazepines are relatively safe medications regarding their interactions with other drugs, but there are some potentially troublesome interactions to keep in mind. For example, concurrent benzodiazepine use increases the blood levels of digitalis and might necessitate downward adjustment in the dose of digitalis; in contrast, antacid use can decrease the absorption of benzodiazepines, and cimetidine delays their clearance (Baldessarini 1985). Finally, alcohol and benzodiazepines have a potentiating effect that can lead to quick intoxication, even with small amounts of alcohol, in an elderly patient who is using benzodiazepines on a long-term basis.

Respiratory Depression and Other Breathing Problems

Many elderly patients with chronic obstructive pulmonary disease (COPD) also manifest impaired quality of sleep (Guilleminault 1990). Hypnotic benzodiazepines are often prescribed on a long-term basis to these patients despite documentation that benzodiazepines can cause hypoventilation in patients with severe COPD (Geddes et al. 1976). Another important issue that is somewhat ignored in the literature is the deleterious effect of benzodiazepines on sleep-related breathing disorders. Guilleminault (1990) points out that chronic usage of these medications can lead to obstructive sleep apnea in elderly subjects who are chronic snorers. In addition, it appears that hypnotic benzodiazepine use in postmyocardial infarction patients for 3 to 6 months may lead to repetitive short central apneas that are accompanied by brief, more marked decreases in oxygen saturation. These findings suggest the need for caution when prescribing benzodiazepines to elderly patients with respiratory problems.

Abuse, Dependence, and Withdrawal

As noted previously, there is sufficient evidence now to establish that benzodiazepines can be habit-forming (Burch 1990; Grantham 1987), although some clinicians contend that abuse of these medications is mostly limited to patients with substance abuse problems (Uhlenhuth et al. 1988; Woods et al. 1988). Physical dependence has been reported even when these medications are taken at doses within the clinical range over a period of time (Rickels et al. 1988; Uhlenhuth et al. 1988). There are conflicting reports, however, as to what length of exposure to these medications can give rise to dependence and withdrawal. There is evidence of withdrawal after 4 to 6 weeks of diazepam therapy (Murphy et al. 1984). On the other hand, no such evidence was found by Rickels et al. (1983) after 6 weeks of treatment with diazepam in new patients.

There are strong suggestions, however, that the risk of physical dependence on benzodiazepines increases substantially after regular usage for more than 6 months (Rickels et al. 1988), with approximately 40% of patients using benzodiazepines beyond 8 months manifesting withdrawal on discontinuation. Alprazolam seems to lead to the worst withdrawal response, possibly because of alprazolam's high affinity for benzodiazepine receptors (Ayd 1988; Dickinson et al. 1990). Signs and symptoms of withdrawal from benzodiazepines are listed in Table 5-3.

Most elderly subjects can be tapered off benzodiazepines on an outpatient basis if certain guidelines are followed (see Table 5-4). In some cases in which the usage has been very long-term and possibly complicated by other medical illnesses, it may be advisable to hospitalize the patient. Posthospital follow-up can be organized with an emphasis on education of patients and family members while working very closely with the primary physicians. Emotional support and strengthening of social systems can be very helpful.

Alternative Management Strategies for Anxiety and Insomnia

Alternative interventions for anxiety can consist of both pharmacological and nonpharmacological management strategies. For anxiety, aza-pirones, a new class of psychotherapeutic drugs, seem to show promise. Buspirone is the prototype of these compounds and the only one thus far approved for use in the United States. It is an anxiolytic with partial serotonin-agonist properties that appears to have an efficacy comparable to that of diazepam in patients with generalized anxiety disorder (Rickels et al. 1982). Buspirone's nonaddictive profile and an absence of with-

Table 5–3.   Benzodiazepine withdrawal syndrome

Mild	Severe
Elevated pulse and respiration rates	Extreme agitation
Apprehension and irritability	Emotional incontinence
Coarse tremors and shaking	Auditory or visual hallucinations
Hyperreflexia	Hyperthermia
Hot flushes and sweating	Delirium
Nausea and anorexia	Paranoid psychosis
Rebound anxiety and insomnia	Generalized convulsions

Table 5–4.   Guidelines for withdrawing elderly outpatients from benzodiazepines

Educate the patient about signs and symptoms of withdrawal.
Substitute longer-acting benzodiazepines for shorter-acting ones.
Withdraw at a rate of 5%–10% every 3–5 days.
Be prepared to modify your withdrawal regime when indicated.
Closely monitor patient's progress.
Institute nonpharmacological therapies for anxiety and insomnia when appropriate.
Be supportive and empathic during the period of withdrawal.

drawal symptoms when discontinuing treatment seem to show its advantages over benzodiazepines in treating chronic anxiety conditions (Rickels et al. 1988).

Unlike benzodiazepines, buspirone does not appear to cause drowsiness, cognitive impairment, psychomotor impairment, or ataxia, even with long-term usage (Smiley and Moskowitz 1986). Preliminary, nonplacebo-controlled studies in geriatric populations indicate that it is well-tolerated, does not cause adverse effects when co-prescribed with a variety of other medications (including antihypertensives, cardiac glycosides, and bronchodilators), and is effective for remediation of chronic anxiety symptoms in these populations (Napoliello 1986). It also appears that in both acute and chronic dosing, the pharmacokinetics of buspirone in the elderly are very similar to those of younger people (Gammans et al. 1989). Such a profile seems to suggest that buspirone may be a particularly desirable anxiolytic for the elderly, especially in situations in which a long-term use is indicated. Some suggestions on the nonpharmacological management of anxiety and sleep disorders in the elderly are given in Table 5-5.

Conclusions

There is ample evidence in the literature of widespread, at times inappropriate, long-term consumption of benzodiazepines by the elderly, primarily for insomnia and anxiety. Findings from the literature suggest that the elderly may be particularly vulnerable to several complications associated with such a usage pattern, including drowsiness, cognitive decline, psychomotor impairment, increased risk of falling, and hip fractures.

Table 5–5.   Nonpharmacological interventions for treatment of anxiety and insomnia

Anxiety
Traditional psychotherapy
Cognitive-behavioral therapies
Relaxation training
Cognitive restructuring
Exposure

Insomnia
Schedule regular hours for bedtime and waking up.
Do not nap during the day.
Exercise lightly every day to keep physically fit and improve the quality of sleep. Do not exercise within a few hours of sleep.
Take dinner at least 2 hours before going to bed.
Keep the bedroom clean and quiet, with a comfortable bed, and use it primarily for sleeping.
Avoid caffeine, nicotine, and any medications with stimulants several hours before going to sleep.
If necessary, help induce sleep by taking a warm bath, having a glass of warm milk, and/or doing light reading.

Source.   Adapted from Sheikh 1991.

Several professional and regulatory agencies in the United States and abroad have strived to provide guidelines for judicious benzodiazepene use. For example, the American Psychiatric Association (1985) recommends a review in patients for whom benzodiazepines are prescribed for more than 3 months. The Committee on the Review of Medicines in the United Kingdom in 1980 recommended that benzodiazepine hypnotics among the elderly be prescribed "for short periods of time, and only after careful consideration" (p. 911). More recently, the Committee on Safety of Medicines (1988) advised against use of benzodiazepine hypnotics for longer than 4 weeks.

The issue of duration of usage is somewhat more difficult to determine in the area of anxiety. For example, many of the anxiety disorders, including generalized anxiety disorder and panic disorder, are chronic in nature, and one may have to choose between no treatment, nonpharmacological treatments, buspirone, and benzodiazepines. The decision can get more complicated when a patient has already been taking benzodiazepines for a few years, reports relief of symptoms, is unwilling to consider any other treatment, and seems to be showing no manifest signs of cognitive deficits or psychomotor impairment. In situations like this, the therapeutic decision hinges on a careful analysis of the clinical condition and risks and benefits of medications. Finally, it is important for clinicians to be knowledgeable about various alternative treatments, both pharmacological and nonpharmacological.

References

American Psychiatric Association, Committee on Peer Review: Manual of Psychiatric Peer Review, 3rd Edition. Washington, DC, American Psychiatric Association, 1985

Ashton H: Adverse effects of prolonged benzodiazepine use. Adverse Drug Reaction Bulletin 118:440–443, 1986

Ayd FJ: Problems associated with alprazolam therapy. International Drug Therapy Newsletter 23:29–31, 1988

Baldessarini RJ: Chemotherapy in Psychiatry: Principles and Practice, Revised and Enlarged Edition. Cambridge, MA, Harvard University Press, 1985

Balter MB, Manheimer DI, Mellinger GD, et al: A cross-national comparison of anti-anxiety/sedative drug use. Curr Med Res Opin 8 (suppl 4):5–20, 1984

Blazer D, George L, Hughes D: The epidemiology of anxiety disorders: an age comparison, in Anxiety Disorders in the Elderly. Edited by Salzman C, Liebowitz B. New York, Springer, 1991, pp 17–30

Bo O, Haffner O, Langard O, et al: Ethanol and diazepam as causative agents in road accidents, in Alcohol, Drugs, and Traffic Safety. Edited by Iraelstam S, Lambert S. Toronto, Addiction Research Foundation of Toronto, 1975, pp 439–448

Boston Collaborative Drug Surveillance Program: Clinical depression of the nervous system due to diazepam and chlordiazepoxide in relation to cigarette smoking and age. N Engl J Med 288:277–280, 1973

Burch EA Jr: Use and misuse of benzodiazepines in the elderly. Psychiatr Med 8(2):97–105, 1990

Committee on Safety of Medicines: Benzodiazepines: dependence and withdrawal symptoms (Study No 21). Committee on Safety of Medicines, January 1988

Committee on the Review of Medicines: Systematic review of the benzodiazepines. Br Med J 280:910–912, 1980

Craik FIM: Age differences in human memory, in Handbook of the Psychology of Human Aging. Edited by Birren JE, Schaie KW. New York, Van Nostrand Reinhold, 1977, pp 384–420

Cutler NR, Narang PK: Implications of dosing tricyclic antidepressants and benzodiazepines in geriatrics. Psychiatr Clin North Am 7:845–861, 1984

Dickinson B, Rush PA, Radcliffe AB: Alprazolam use and dependence: a retrospective analysis of 30 cases of withdrawal. West J Med 152:604–608, 1990

Gammans RE, Westrick ML, Shea JP, et al: Pharmacokinetics of buspirone in elderly subjects. J Clin Pharmacol 29:72–78, 1989

Geddes DM, Rudolf M, Saunders KB: Effect of nitrazepam and flurazepam on the ventilatory response to carbon dioxide. Thorax 31:548–551, 1976

Gottlieb GL: Sleep disorders and their management: special considerations in the elderly. Am J Med 88 (suppl 3A):29S–33S, 1990

Granek P, Baker SP, Abbey H, et al: Medication and diagnoses in relation to falls in a long-term care facility. J Am Geriatr Soc 35:503–511, 1987

Grantham P: Benzodiazepine abuse. Br J Hosp Med 37:292–300, 1987

Greenblatt DJ, Allen MD: Toxicity of nitrazepam in the elderly: a report from the Boston Collaborative Drug Surveillance Program. Br J Clin Pharmacol 5:407–413, 1978

Greenblatt DJ, Divoll M, Harmatz JS, et al: Kinetics and clinical effects of flurazepam in young and elderly noninsomniacs. Clin Pharmacol Ther 30:475–486, 1981

Greenblatt DJ, Divoll M, Abernethy DR, et al: Alprazolam kinetics in the elderly: relation to antipyrine disposition. Arch Gen Psychiatry 40:287–290, 1983

Greenblatt DJ, Shader RI, Harmatz JS: Implications of altered drug disposition in the elderly: studies of benzodiazepines. J Clin Pharmacol 29:866–872, 1989

Guilleminault C: Benzodiazepines, breathing, and sleep. Am J Med 88 (suppl 3A):25S–28S, 1990

Hershey LA, Kim KY: Diagnosis and treatment of anxiety in the elderly. Rational Drug Therapy 22(1):3–6, 1988

Hindmarch I, Clyde CA: The effects of triazolam and nitrazepam on sleep quality, morning vigilance and psychomotor performance. Arzneimittel-Forschung 30:1163–1166, 1980

Kanto J, Kangas L, Aaltonen L, et al: Effect of age on the pharmacokinetics and sedative effect of flunitrazepam. Int J Clin Pharmacol Ther Toxicol 19:400–404, 1981

Kroboth PD, McAuley JW, Smith RB: Alprazolam in the elderly: pharmacokinetics and pharmacodynamics during multiple dosing. Psychopharmacology 100:477–484, 1990

Lader MH, Petursson H: Benzodiazepine derivatives—side effects and dangers. Biol Psychiatry 16:1195–2021, 1981

Lavizzo-Mourey R: Preventing adverse drug reactions in the elderly, in Practicing Prevention for the Elderly. Edited by Lavizzo-Mourey R, Day SC, Diserens D, et al. Philadelphia, PA, Hanley and Balfus, 1989, pp 47–62

Louis Harris and Associates: Tranquilizers: use and perceived abuse in America (Study No 871031). Louis Harris and Associates, September 1987

Lydiard RB, Laraia MT, Ballenger JC, et al: Emergence of depressive symptoms in patients receiving alprazolam for panic disorder. Am J Psychiatry 144:664–665, 1987

Mellinger GD, Balter MB, Uhlenhuth EH: Prevalence and correlates of the long-term regular use of anxiolytics. JAMA 251:375–379, 1984

Moran MG, Thompson TL II, Nies AS: Sleep disorders in the elderly. Am J Psychiatry 145:1369–1378, 1988

Morgan K, Dallosso H, Ebrahim S, et al: Prevalence, frequency, and duration of hypnotic drug use among the elderly living at home. Br Med J 296:601–602, 1988

Murphy P, Hindmarch I, Hyland CM: Aspects of short-term use of two benzodiazepine hypnotics in the elderly. Age Ageing 11:222–228, 1982

Murphy SM, Owen RT, Tyrer PJ: Withdrawal symptoms after six weeks' treatment with diazepam. Lancet 2:1389, 1984

Napoliello MJ: An interim multicenter report on 677 anxious geriatric out-patients treated with buspirone. Br J Clin Pract 40:71–73, 1986

National Disease and Therapeutic Index (NDTI). Ambler, PA, IMS America, 1986

National Institute on Drug Abuse: Drug Abuse Warning Network (DAWN). Statistical series. Rockville, MD, National Institute on Drug Abuse, 1986, ser 1, no 5

Nikaido AM, Ellinwood EH Jr, Heatherly DG, et al: Age-related increase in sensitivity to benzodiazepines as assessed by task difficulty. Psychopharmacology (Berlin) 100:90–97, 1990

Omslander JG: Drug therapy in the elderly. Ann Intern Med 94:711–722, 1981

Oswald I: Insomnia. Br J Hosp Med 31:219–224, 1984

Papper S: Clinical Nephrology. Boston, MA, Little, Brown, 1978

Petursson H, Gudjonsson G, Lader MH: Psychometric performance during chronic benzodiazepine treatment and withdrawal. Psychopharmacology 81:345, 1983

Pomara N, Deptula D, Singh R, et al: Cognitive toxicity of benzodiazepines in the elderly, in Anxiety Disorders in the Elderly. Edited by Salzman CL, Liebowitz B. New York, Springer, 1991, pp 175–196

Ray W, Griffin M, Schaffner W, et al: Psychotropic drug use and the risk of hip fracture. N Engl J Med 316:363–369, 1987

Ray WA, Griffin MR, Downey W: Benzodiazepines of long and short half-life and the risk of hip fracture. JAMA 262:3303–3307, 1989

Reidenberg MM, Levy M, Warner H, et al: Relationship between diazepam dose, plasma level, age, and central nervous system depression. Clin Pharmacol Ther 23:371–374, 1978

Rickels K, Weisman K, Norstad N, et al: Buspirone and diazepam in anxiety: a controlled study. J Clin Psychiatry 43(12, sec 2):81–86, 1982

Rickels K, Case G, Downing RW, et al: Long-term diazepam therapy and clinical outcome. JAMA 250:767–771, 1983

Rickels K, Schweizer E, Csanalosi I, et al: Long-term treatment of anxiety and risk of withdrawal: prospective comparison of clorazepate and buspirone. Arch Gen Psychiatry 45:444–450, 1988

Rosenbaum J: Anxiety, in Outpatient Psychiatry. Edited by Lazare A. Baltimore, MD, Williams & Wilkins, 1979, pp 252–256

Rowe JW, Besdine R: Drug therapy, in Health and Disease in Old Age. Edited by Rowe JW, Besdine RW. Boston, MA, Little, Brown, 1982, pp 39–53

Shaw SM, Opit LJ: Need for supervision in the elderly receiving long-term prescribed medication. Br Med J 1:505–507, 1976

Sheikh JI: Anxiety disorders in the elderly, in Current Problems in Geriatrics. Edited by Blazer DG, Hazzard WR. Littleton, MA, Mosby–Year Book, February 1991

Skegg DCG, Richards SM, Doll R: Minor tranquillisers and road accidents. Br Med J 1:917–919, 1979

Smiley A, Moskowitz H: Effects of long-term administration of buspirone and diazepam on driver steering control. Am J Med 80 (suppl 3b):22–29, 1986

Sobel KG, McCart GM: Drug use and accidental falls in an intermediate care facility. Drug Intelligence and Clinical Pharmacy 17:539–542, 1983

Sorock GS, Shimkin EE: Benzodiazepine sedatives and the risk of falling in a community-dwelling elderly cohort. Arch Intern Med 148:2441–2444, 1988

Stephens RC, Haney CA, Underwood S: Drug taking among the elderly, in Treatment Research Report and Monograph Series, National Institute on Drug Abuse (DHHS Publ No ADM-83-1229). Washington, DC, U.S. Government Printing Office, 1982, pp 7–25

Sussman N: The benzodiazepines: selection and use in treating anxiety, insomnia and other disorders. Hospital Formulary 20:298–305, 1985

Sussman N, Chou JCY: Current issues in benzodiazepine use for anxiety disorders. Psychiatric Annals 18:139–145, 1988

Taylor JL, Tinklenberg JR: Cognitive impairment and benzodiazepines, in Psychopharmacology: The Third Generation of Progress. Edited by Meltzer HY. New York, Raven, 1987, pp 1449–1454

Uhlenhuth EH, DeWit H, Balter MB, et al: Risks and benefits of long-term benzodiazepine use. J Clin Psychopharmacol 8:161–167, 1988

Warren R: Drugs in fatally injured drivers in the province of Ontario, in Alcohol, Drugs, and Traffic Safety, Vol 1. Edited by Goldberg L. Stockholm, Almquist and Wiskell, 1981

Williamson J, Chopin JM: Adverse reactions to prescribed drugs in the elderly: a multicentre investigation. Age Ageing 9:73–80, 1980

Woods JH, Katz JL, Winger G, et al: Use and abuse of benzodiazepines: issues relevant to prescribing. JAMA 260:3476–3480, 1988

Chapter 6

Efficacy and Side Effects of Cholinergic Drugs Used in the Treatment of Alzheimer's Disease

Vinod Kumar, M.D., M.R.C.Psych.
Michel Calache, M.D.

*D*ementia of the Alzheimer type (DAT) is a neurodegenerative disorder affecting several neurotransmitter systems of the brain (Rossor et al. 1984; Roth and Wischik 1985). The cholinergic system deficit, the most widely studied, has been reported to be associated with the memory problems of DAT patients (Coyle et al. 1983; Whitehouse et al. 1982). Cholinergic deficit in these patients appears to consist of reduction in 1) acetylcholine synthesis, 2) choline acetyltransferase (CAT) activity, and 3) choline uptake (Davies and Maloney 1976; Perry et al. 1977; Sims et al. 1983). Correction of the cholinergic deficit has produced only mild and inconsistent improvement in the cognitive functions of DAT patients.

There have been four strategies to correct cholinergic deficits in DAT patients: 1) precursor loading, 2) the use of cholinesterase inhibitors, 3) the combination of precursor loading and cholinesterase inhibitors, and 4) the administration of muscarinic and nicotinic cholinergic agonists (Kumar and Becker 1989). However, none of these strategies has produced a dramatic clinical change in the cognitive function and associated behavior deficits in DAT patients. There are some practical problems in using cholinergic drugs because of their relatively short duration of action and the occurrence of some disabling side effects. To summarize this complex problem, we will discuss these four strategies independently, including efficacy and side effects of various cholinergic drugs used to date in the treatment of DAT patients.

Precursor Loading

Precursor loading aims to increase the synthesis and release of acetylcholine in the synaptic terminals. The brain does not have the necessary enzymes to synthesize choline de novo (Cohen and Wurtman 1976). Exogenously administered precursors may, however, help increase acetylcholine synthesis (Vroulis et al. 1981). Both choline and phosphatidylcholine (lecithin) are acetylcholine precursors. Lecithin is a source of choline and has similar physiological effects (Wood and Allison 1982). Oral choline is not an ideal precursor of acetylcholine because the compound is quickly cleared from plasma and tissues and consequently the period of effectiveness is limited (Wood and Allison 1982). Oral lecithin provides a longer acting and better tolerated precursor of choline (Wurtman et al. 1977).

Choline uptake is probably the rate-limiting step in the biosynthesis of acetylcholine (Haubrich and Chippendale 1977). The uptake mechanism occurs via a sodium-dependent, high-affinity transport system. This system is saturated under normal conditions. There are certain authors who believe that under conditions of increased neuronal demand, choline can be taken up by a second low-affinity uptake system (Jenike et al. 1986). If this is true, increased precursor availability may increase acetylcholine synthesis.

The concomitant administration of choline and agents that enhance the utilization of exogenously administered precursors has also been tested. These *nootropic* or extraneuronal metabolic enhancers facilitate transmembrane influx and increase carbohydrate metabolism. Other drugs, such as 4-aminopyridine, facilitate transmembrane calcium influx and may increase choline uptake and acetylcholine synthesis. Preclinical tests have suggested that these agents can induce an increase in acetylcholine concentration in the brain (Cohen and Wurtman 1975, 1976). However, clinical trials have not shown evidence of altered spontaneous release of acetylcholine.

These presynaptic approaches have the advantage of mimicking the phasic action of cholinergic cells, but at the same time they require the presence of intact neurons to be effective (Mohs et al. 1979). In an interesting study by Sullivan et al. (1982), 12 patients were given physostigmine. It was found that a favorable response to physostigmine could not predict a favorable response to lecithin in a second experiment with these same patients.

The Acetylcholine Precursors Choline and Lecithin

Efficacy. Choline and lecithin have been tested extensively in DAT patients. We reviewed 21 clinical trials of choline and lecithin in these patients (see Table 6-1). Nine studies evaluated the effect of choline, and 12 evaluated the effect of lecithin. Thirteen were double-blind trials, and the remainder were open clinical trials. Only a few studies reported positive results. Among the few positive reports, Vroulis et al. (1981) found the most significant improvement with their patients. In a double-blind, placebo-controlled design, 18 patients received 70 g of lecithin for 2 to 8 days. Nine of these patients (50%) were reported to improve. Dysken et al. (1982b) conducted a double-blind, placebo-controlled trial of lecithin to test its effects on the cognition of five patients with early dementia. The authors found a significant improvement in both auditory and visual presentation on a word recognition task at 15 g of lecithin per day. Fovall et al. (1980) found similar improvement for auditory and visual word recognition with the same dose (12 g) of choline per day.

On the other hand, Weintraub et al. (1983) did not find any improvement in their patients but reported a slowing in the degree of deterioration over a 6-month period in comparison with patients who did not receive lecithin. However, several other studies have reported either no effect or worsening of the cognitive functions with administration of lecithin and choline (Table 6-1). In one study (Little et al. 1985), poor compliers (i.e., those who consistently took less than 75% of the prescribed dose) did better on verbal learning and self-care than did good compliers, which suggests a therapeutic optimal dose (i.e., "therapeutic window") for the effects of lecithin. This may explain the negative results of several studies. Nine double-blind studies (two with choline and seven with lecithin) reported no benefit from the use of choline or lecithin in improving the cognitive functions of DAT patients (Bajada 1982; Brinkman et al. 1982; Domino et al. 1982; Dysken et al. 1982a, 1982b; Heyman et al. 1982; Little et al. 1985; Peters and Levine 1979; Smith et al. 1978). These studies included 95 patients with DAT who had been receiving a dose range of 8.3 to 19.0 g per day for an average of 6.5 days. In two studies (Ferris et al. 1982; Jenike et al. 1986), the metabolic enhancers piracetam and ergoloid mesylates were used in conjunction with precursor loading. The addition of metabolic enhancers did not lead to a dramatic improvement in the cognitive function of these patients.

However, the addition of piracetam to choline did lead to some improvement in a very small number of subjects (4 out of 15), but there was no change when ergoloid mesylate, instead of piracetam, was used in conjunction with choline.

Side effects. The side effects of choline and lecithin in DAT patients have been largely underreported. Most studies reviewed did not report either the presence or the absence of side effects. In general, cholinergic drugs can cause systemic and psychiatric adverse reactions and subclinical laboratory abnormalities. Gastrointestinal disturbances have been the most commonly reported side effects. Other side effects include nausea, decreased appetite, stomach cramps, and diarrhea (Boyd et al. 1977; Domino et al. 1982; Etienne et al. 1978a, 1978b). Systemic adverse reactions include lowered blood pressure (Boyd et al. 1977), dizziness (Dysken et al. 1982b), weight gain (Heyman et al. 1982), and bad skin smell (Etienne et al. 1978b). (The latter side effect has been reported with choline, but not with lecithin.) Psychiatric side effects did not appear de novo. However, two authors reported the worsening of preexisting symptoms. Etienne et al. (1978b) reported increased suspiciousness in one of their patients, and Smith et al. (1978) reported increased depression in a depressive patient. Lecithin was also found to decrease cholesterol-triglyceride ratios (Vroulis et al. 1981).

Cholinesterase Inhibitors

There has been some evidence that choline uptake, even in DAT, is a saturated transport mechanism (Glen et al. 1981). This finding suggests that effective treatment of DAT will require a drug that acts synaptically or postsynaptically. One such approach has been the potentiation of residual cholinergic function by the inhibition of acetyl cholinesterase activity by cholinesterase inhibitors, such as physostigmine and tacrine (tetrahydroaminoacridine [THA]). However, both short- and long-acting cholinesterase inhibitors are drugs with potentially serious side effects that limit their utility as therapeutic agents.

Physostigmine (a short-acting inhibitor) has been shown to reverse scopolamine-induced cognitive deficit. Clinical experience with physostigmine indicates that it can be administered relatively safely in low doses, is easily absorbed, and enters the brain (Thal et al. 1986). One

Table 6–1. Effects of choline and lecithin in patients with dementia of the Alzheimer type

Author (year)	Substance	Study	Number of patients	Age (years)	Daily dose (g)	Duration	Effect on memory	Side effects
Boyd et al. (1977)	Choline chloride	Pilot open clinical trial	7	70–80	5–10	2–4 weeks	0	Nausea, diarrhea, ↓ BP
Etienne et al. (1978a)	Lecithin	Open clinical trial	7	42–81	8	4 weeks	+	↓ in appetite without ↓ in weight
Etienne et al. (1978b)	Choline chloride	Case series	3	76–88	9	4 weeks	0	Bad skin smell, ↑ in suspiciousness
Signoret et al. (1978)	Choline citrate	Open clinical trial	8	59–78	25	4 weeks	+	None
Smith et al. (1978)	Choline bitartrate	Double-blind, placebo-controlled	10	Mean = 77	9	2 weeks	0	↑ in depression in a depressed patient
Mohs et al. (1979)	Choline chloride	Open clinical trial	8	64–86	16	1 week	0	NR
Peters and Levin (1979)	Lecithin	Randomized double-blind	5	58–79	3.6	1 day	0	NR
Renvoize and Jerram (1979)	Choline	Open clinical trial	18	57–84	15	2 months	0	NR

Table 6-1 (continued)

Author (year)	Substance	Study	Number of patients	Age (years)	Daily dose (g)	Duration	Effect on memory	Side effects
Fovall et al. (1980)	Choline bitartrate	Double-blind, placebo-controlled	5	55–71	12	2 months	+	NR
Vroulis et al. (1981)	Lecithin	Double-blind, placebo-controlled, crossover	18	NR	70	2–8 days	+	↓ in cholesterol-triglyceride ratios
Bajada (1982)	Choline chloride	Double-blind crossover	6	Mean = 69	6	1 week	0	NR
Brinkman et al. (1982)	Lecithin	Double-blind crossover	10	65–82	35	2 weeks	0	NR
Domino et al. (1982)	Lecithin	Double-blind, placebo-controlled	20	NR	100	2 weeks	0	Gastrointestinal discomfort
Dysken et al. (1982a, b)	Lecithin	Double-blind crossover	10	54–78	15–30	2–8 weeks	0	NR
Ferris et al. (1982)	Choline; Choline and piracetam	Double-blind crossover	112 15	60–85 60–85	12 9 choline + 8 piracetam	12 weeks 1 week	+	NR

Study	Treatment	Design	N	Age	Dose	Duration	Effect	Side effects
Heyman et al. (1982)	Lecithin	Double-blind crossover	18	59–69	25–40	8 weeks	0	Mild nausea, stomach cramps, dizziness, anorexia, weight gain
Kaye et al. (1982)	Lecithin	Pilot random trial with placebo, THA, and THA + lecithin	10	51–71	60	1 day	0	NR
Sullivan et al. (1982)	Lecithin	Double-blind crossover	8	54–78	20–30	5 weeks	0	NR
Pomara et al. (1983)	Lecithin	Open clinical trial	6	62–82	15	Single dose	0	Occasional diarrhea
Weintraub et al. (1983)	Lecithin	Double-blind crossover	13	54–81	16–20	9 weeks	+	NR
Little et al. (1985)	Lecithin	Double-blind, placebo-controlled	18	Mean = 76	20–25	26 weeks	0	NR

Note. 0 = No effect or a very equivocal effect; + = small improvement; NR = not reported; BP = blood pressure; THA = tacrine.

disadvantage of the drug is that its half-life in plasma is only about 30 minutes (Whelpton 1981), thus limiting its clinical usefulness.

Tetrahydroaminoacridine is another potent centrally acting anticholinesterase inhibitor that has a pharmacological action similar to that of physostigmine. THA is a reversible cholinesterase inhibitor with a much longer duration of action than physostigmine.

Efficacy

Physostigmine. Physostigmine has been the most widely tested drug in DAT patients. It has been mostly used orally or intravenously, but the subcutaneous and intramuscular routes have also been investigated (see Table 6-2). The intravenous route has the advantage of bypassing the gastrointestinal and hepatic pathways. However, only the acute single-dose experimental design has been practicable. Thus the long-term efficacy of physostigmine can only be tested with the oral administration of the drug over an extended period of time.

Using the intravenous method, marked improvement of memory function in selected memory tasks was reported in four double-blind clinical trials (Davis et al. 1979; Johns et al. 1985; Peters and Levin 1979; Sullivan et al. 1982), but in two double-blind studies (Christie et al. 1981; Elble et al. 1988) no effect on memory was reported. Elble et al. (1988) used a relatively high dose of physostigmine; some of their patients received physostigmine at 900 mg/m^2 of body surface area by intravenous infusion over 2.25 hours.

Studies of the effects of physostigmine using the oral, subcutaneous, and intramuscular routes have been less encouraging. Only two (Peters and Levin 1982; Stern et al. 1988) out of a total of eight double-blind studies listed in Table 6-2 showed marked improvement. These two studies have shown this improvement with relatively high doses of orally administered physostigmine (9–14.5 mg). Five studies administered physostigmine to 40 patients for 2 months or more (2 months to 3.5 years) (Beller et al. 1988; Jotkowitz 1983; Mayeux et al. 1987; Peters and Levin 1982; Thal et al. 1989). In four of these studies (Beller et al. 1988; Mayeux et al. 1987; Peters and Levin 1982; Thal et al. 1989) marked or moderate improvement was reported, while in the remaining study (Jotkowitz 1983) there was no effect. The results of these studies of chronic administration have been much better than the results obtained from studies involving the acute oral administration of physostigmine. In summary, most of the trials of physostigmine have been marginally successful and without meaningful clinical improvement.

Tacrine (tetrahydroaminoacridine). Recently, several studies have reported rather promising results with THA. Summers et al. (1986) reported that 17 DAT patients who participated in a three-phase study showed dramatic improvement when given THA in combination with lecithin. Significant improvement was observed in their global assessment, their orientation, and their results on the name-learning test. Nyback et al. (1988) reported the results of an open study involving 10 DAT patients who were given THA 25 to 200 mg/day. Five of the 10 patients (50%) showed a measurable improvement in their cognitive function (verbal ability and memory) and in their behavior. Similar results have also been reported by Levy (1988), who in the open phase studied the effects of THA on 6 DAT patients. Three of them (50%) showed improvement in cognitive functioning and activities of daily living. In summary, in seven out of nine studies on the use of THA in DAT patients, measurable improvement has been reported, while in the two remaining studies (Fitten et al. 1988; Kaye et al. 1982) no significant improvement in the patients was found (Table 6-3). However, both of these studies used THA for a very short duration—Kaye et al. (1982) for 1 day and Fitten et al. (1988) for 1 week only.

Becker et al. (in press) have reported that a very long-acting cholinesterase inhibitor, metrifonate, may have some promise in the treatment of DAT. Preliminary results involving 20 patients indicate that this drug, when given once a week, appears to maintain a moderate degree of inhibition of cholinesterase enzymes while having virtually no intolerable side effects. The efficacy study is still in progress.

Side Effects

Physostigmine. The side effects of physostigmine in DAT patients have been underreported. Eighteen of the 32 studies reviewed failed to report either the presence or absence of side effects. Most studies involving intravenous administration of physostigmine used a single or one-day dose of 0.15–1 mg physostigmine. Peters and Levin (1979) and Elble et al. (1988) reported the presence of nausea with physostigmine at doses of 0.15 mg intravenously and 900 mg/m^2 body surface area, respectively.

Table 6–2. Effects of physostigmine in patients with dementia of the Alzheimer type

Author (year)	Study	Number of patients	Age (years)	Daily dose (mg)	Duration	Effect on memory	Side effects
Oral administration							
Bajada (1982)	Double-blind crossover	6	Mean = 69	2.4	1 week	–	NR
Caltagirone et al. (1982)	Open clinical trial	8	NR	4	1 month	–	NR
Peters and Levin (1982)	Double-blind, controlled	9	54–79	9	3–18 months	+++	Nausea
Jotkowitz (1983)	Open clinical trial	10	65–80	10–15	10 months	0	None
Thal and Fuld (1983)	Open clinical trial	12	NR	3–16	2 days	+++	Nausea, vomiting, sweating, queasiness
Thal et al. (1983)	Open clinical trial followed by double-blind crossover	8	57–78	3–16	6–8 days	+	NR
Wettstein (1983)	Double-blind single crossover	8	50–70	3–10	2–6 weeks	–	Nausea, diarrhea

Muramoto et al. (1984)	Open clinical trial	1	Mean = 62	1–3	Acute	++	NR
Beller et al. (1985)	Double-blind multiple crossover	8	NR	7–14	2 days	0	Tachycardia, hypertensive episode, euphoria
Mohs et al. (1985)	Open clinical trial	12	52–76	0.5–2.0	14–19 days	0	NR
Beller et al. (1988)	Open trial with long-term administration	5	NR	7	1–3.75 years	++	None
Thal et al. (1986)	Double-blind	16	NR	4–16	2 weeks	0	NR
Mayeux et al. (1987)	Case reports	2	62 + 76	4–14	4–8 weeks	++	Muscle jerks, myoclonus
Stern et al. (1988)	Double-blind crossover	14	Mean = 68.8	14.5	5–6 weeks	+++	Nausea, sweating, cramps, fatigue, ↓ in appetite, palpitations, dizziness, diarrhea
Thal et al. (1989)	Double-blind	5	56–80	4.16	3 months	++	Dizziness

Table 6–2 (continued)

Author (year)	Study	Number of patients	Age (years)	Daily dose (mg)	Duration	Effect on memory	Side effects
Subcutaneous administration							
Smith and Swash (1979)	Case report	1	Mean = 42	1	Acute	0	NR
Wettstein (1983)	Double-blind single crossover	8	50–70	0.01–0.02 mg/kg	12 weeks	–	Nausea, diarrhea
Intramuscular administration							
Muramoto et al. (1979)	Double-blind	1	Mean = 57	1	Acute	++	NR
Peters and Levin (1979)	Double-blind	5	58–79	0.005–0.015 mg/kg	Acute	++	None
Smith et al. (1982)	Clinical open trial	3	41–50	0.8–1.0	Acute	0	Exacerbation of mild parkinsonian features
Schwartz and Kohlstaedt (1986)	Double-blind	11	61–83	0.004–0.3 mg/kg	Acute	0	NR
Intravenous administration							
Davis et al. (1979)	Double-blind	6	Mean = 64	0.125–5.0	Acute	+++	NR

Study	Design	N	Age	Dose	Acute	Effect	Nausea
Peters and Levin (1979)	Double-blind	5	58–79	0.15	Acute	+++	Nausea
Christie et al. (1981)	Double-blind	11	NR	0.25–1.0	Acute	0	NR
Davis and Mohs (1982)	Open clinical trial	6	Mean = 64	0.125–0.5	Acute	+++	NR
Sullivan et al. (1982)	Double-blind	12	51–72	0.25–0.5	Acute	+++	NR
Agnoli et al. (1983)	Open clinical trial	10	54–73	1	Acute	+	NR
Muramoto et al. (1984)	Open clinical trial	4	51–63	1–3	Acute	+	NR
Johns et al. (1985)	Double-blind	20	NR	0.125–0.5	Acute	+++	NR
Blackwood and Christie (1986)	Open clinical trial	12	54–68	0.375–0.75	Acute	+	NR
Rose and Moulthrop (1986)	Case report	1	Mean = 79	0.125–5.0	Acute	+	NR
Elble et al. (1988)	Double-blind	16	55–81	0.3–0.9 per m^2 surface area	Acute	0	Gastrointestinal disturbances, nausea, lightheadedness, abdominal cramps

Note. − = negative effect; 0 = no effect or very equivocal effect; + = mild improvement; ++ = moderate improvement or unclear effect in some memory functions; +++ = marked improvement, especially in relation to selected memory functions; NR = no response; Acute = single dose or multiple single doses.

Administration of physostigmine by oral, subcutaneous, and intramuscular routes produced the same types of side effects: namely, nausea, vomiting, diaphoresis, tachycardia, euphoria, and an exacerbation of mild parkinsonian features. Studies involving chronic rather than acute oral administration of physostigmine have frequently reported various side effects, including nausea, vomiting, muscle jerks, and myoclonus. Among 25 studies with acute doses of physostigmine, as well as in doses given for less than 8 weeks duration, side effects were reported in only 6 of them. Of the 7 studies of chronic administration (i.e., physostigmine given for more than 8 consecutive weeks, side effects were reported in 4. One of these studies (Beller et al. 1988) reported no side effects in patients receiving 7 mg/day of physostigmine for 1–3.75 years; however, this open trial included only five patients. The underreported adverse reactions in several of these studies make it difficult to derive conclusions about the frequency of side effects experienced by patients following physostigmine administration. However, there appears to be a direct relationship between the dose and the severity of the reported side effects.

Tacrine (tetrahydroaminoacridine).   Fifty to eighty percent of patients on THA have reported experiencing various side effects (Kumar 1988). Summers et al. (1981), in an open trial, reported that 33% of patients experienced nausea and diaphoresis. Emesis was induced in 16% of patients after the single intravenous administration of 0.5–1 mg/kg of THA. Kaye et al. (1982) conducted the first double-blind study of THA. They did not report any side effects, but they used very small doses of THA (30 mg/day). Among the nine studies that we summarized in Table 6-3, four (Nyback et al. 1988; Summers et al. 1981, 1986; Wilcock et al. 1988) reported gastrointestinal disturbances, including nausea, belching, vomiting, abdominal discomfort, and diarrhea.

The most problematic side effect has been the elevation of liver enzymes—namely, aspartate transaminase, serum glutamic-oxaloacetic transaminase (SGOT), serum glutamic pyruvic transaminase (SGPT), lactate dehydrogenase, and alkaline phosphatase (Ames et al. 1988; Fitten et al. 1988; Gauthier et al. 1988; Levy 1988; Wilcock et al. 1988). However, these elevations are reversible if the drug is reduced or discontinued (Fitten et al. 1988; Kumar and Becker 1989; Levy 1988). In all of our patients in whom a rise in levels occurred, it took 3 to 5 weeks to have increased levels of SGOT and SGPT, and it took 4 to 6 weeks for these levels to return to the normal range. In one patient (see Figure 6-1), SGOT and SGPT levels started rising in the fifth week. We stopped the THA at this time because of the rise in SGOT and SGPT levels; however, the levels peaked in the sixth week, and it took 5–6 weeks for these levels to return to the normal range. A liver biopsy from one of the patients receiving THA showed a noncaseating epithelioid granulomatous reaction (Ames et al. 1988). In most of the studies in which side effects were reported (Table 6-3), the doses ranged between 25–250 mg of THA given for at least 1 week.

Other reported side effects are delayed cutaneous hypersensitivity reaction and autonomic side effects such as rhinorrhea, hypersalivation, hypotension, sinus bradycardia (40 beat/minute), shivering, increased frequency of micturition, and muscle stiffness. Agitation has been reported in a study with a low dose (25 mg) of THA per day (Wilcock et al. 1988). A United States multicenter study has not reported the details of the side effects other than some reports suggesting that 20% of the patients showed elevated liver enzymes, which returned to a normal range within 5–6 weeks after dose reduction or discontinuation of the medications (Kumar and Becker 1989).

Efficacy of Combined Administration of Cholinesterase Inhibitors and Precursor Loading

Because of the disappointing results obtained from the administration of choline or lecithin alone, and the clinically nonsignificant results obtained with cholinesterase inhibitors, several investigators have given a combination of both treatments in order to increase the treatment response and improve memory. Peters and Levin (1979) compared the effects of physostigmine alone to the effects of a combination of physostigmine and lecithin in five patients with DAT. The authors reported benefit from the combination of both drugs. These patients demonstrated improvement in total recall and decrease in intrusions. These findings have not been confirmed by Wettstein (1983) in a double-blind, single-dose crossover design comparing the effect of placebo with the effect of a combination of 18 g of lecithin and 3–10 mg of orally administered physostigmine. There was no improvement in eight patients with DAT.

Two studies have assessed the effects of chronic administration of both physostigmine and lecithin in DAT patients. One study reported a

Table 6–3. Effects of tacrine (THA) in patients with dementia of the Alzheimer type

Author (year)	Study	Number of patients	Age (years)	Daily dose	Duration	Effect on memory	Side effects
Summers et al. (1981)	Open clinical trial	12	Mean = 72.25 (73–85)	0.5–1.5 mg/kg iv	Single dose	+++	Nausea, diaphoresis
Kaye et al. (1982)	Double-blind	10	51–71	30 mg po	1 day (× 3 doses)	+	NR
Summers et al. (1986)	Phase I: Open clinical trial	17	Mean = 70.65 ± 1.92	25–200 mg THA + lecithin po	7–10 days	++	Nausea, diaphoresis, belching, emesis, abdominal discomfort, diarrhea, increased micturition
	Phase II: Double-blind	14	Mean = 70.65 ± 1.92	25–200 mg THA + lecithin po	3 weeks	+++	NR
	Phase III: Open clinical trial	12		25–200 mg THA + lecithin po	6–12 months	+	NR
Ames et al. (1988)	Case report	1	61	150–200 mg THA; 600 mg lecithin po	14 weeks	++	↑ AT; liver biopsy: non-caseating epithelioid granulomatous reaction; delayed cutaneous hypersensitivity
Fitten et al. (1988)	Phase I: Open clinical trial	10	70.3 ± 4.9	25–250 mg po THA; 30 g/day lecithin (= best dose)	1–2 weeks	0	Sinus bradycardia, nausea, vomiting, diaphoresis, mild enzyme elevation

	Phase II: Double-blind	10				0	
	Phase III						
		6		< 200 mg/day THA po + lecithin (9 g/day)	8 weeks	++	Autonomic side effects; reversible elevations in SGOT, SGPT, LDH, and/or alkaline phosphatase
Gauthier et al. (1988)	Single-blind	51	Mean = 68.5 (53–85)	25–150 mg THA + 1.2 g lecithin po	8 weeks	+++	
Levy (1988)	Double-blind crossover	35 (OP = 6; Co = 29)	NR	150 mg po	NR	NR	Reversible liver toxicity; ↑ AT
Nyback et al. (1988)	Open clinical trial	10	Mean = 63.7	25–200 mg po	1–2 weeks	+	Nausea, vomiting, muscular stiffness
Wilcock et al. (1988)	Open clinical trial	8	NR	25 mg po	NR	NR	Hypotension, sinus bradycardia (40 beats/minute); ↑ liver function indices; mild to severe GI tract disorders; shivering; agitation; increased frequency of micturition

Note. 0 = no improvement; + = mild improvement; ++ = moderate improvement; +++ = marked improvement; NR = not reported; THA = tacrine; AT = aspartate transaminase; SGOT = serum glutamic-oxaloacetic transaminase; SGPT = serum glutamic pyruvic transaminase; LDH = lactate dehydrogenase; OP = open phase; Co = crossover; GI = gastrointestinal.

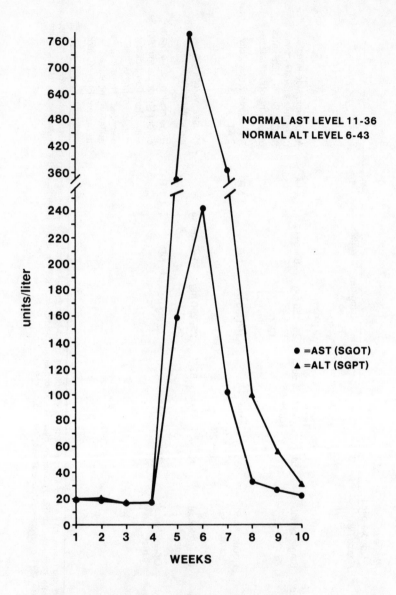

Figure 6-1. Rise in SGOT and SGPT levels in one patient following administration of tacrine (THA) for more than 4 weeks. Medication was stopped after the first report, and it took 5–6 weeks for the levels to return to predrug levels.

beneficial effect of the combined treatment approach in mildly to moderately severe DAT (Peters and Levin 1982). The doses used were 0.5–3.0 mg oral physostigmine and 0.2 g oral lecithin. Another study (Thal et al. 1986) reported no effect on the degree of memory change with the combined physostigmine-lecithin therapy. In this latter study the oral doses were 2–2.5 mg of physostigmine and 10.8 g of lecithin. Another study (Bajada 1982) combined 6 g of choline (instead of lecithin) with 2.4 mg of physostigmine but found that the effect of this combined therapy was no different from that of placebo and from that of each drug given alone.

Kaye et al. (1982), in a double-blind crossover design, gave 30 mg of THA and 60 mg of lecithin orally for a day in four combinations using placebo. They observed no significant improvement in memory functions using a 60-g total dose of lecithin or a 30-mg total dose of THA. However, they found that lecithin in combination with THA facilitated some cognitive functions in the less impaired patients. Gauthier et al. (1988), in a single-blind design, gave 51 DAT patients 25–150 mg of THA and 1.2 g of lecithin. The authors reported a small but measurable and statistically significant improvement in cognitive functions as well as in these patients' activities of daily living. In addition, half of the patients improved in their ability to draw a clock. The patients also improved in their verbal word fluency and on the selective reminding task.

In another double-blind crossover study, 10 patients were given THA (25–250 mg/day) in combination with lecithin for a week. There was no significant difference in placebo and drug-treatment–phase performances on various neuropsychological tests (Fitten et al. 1988). In a more recent study, Fitten et al. (1990) undertook another double-blind trial of orally administered THA and lecithin. No therapeutic effect was evident after 3 weeks of treatment. However, three patients continued long-term treatment with measurable cognitive improvement, while one displayed clinical improvement.

The results of a Canadian double-blind, crossover, multicenter study of THA-lecithin combination treatment have been published (Gauthier et al. 1990). In this study DAT patients were in the intermediate stage of their illness. Initially, 52 patients were recruited for the establishment of efficacy and safety of the drug combination. The doses used were 4.7 g/day of lecithin and up to 100 mg/day of THA. The authors reported no significant improvement on several of the clinical scales.

This question of comparative efficacy of THA plus lecithin versus THA alone is not yet settled; we will have to wait for the reports of several ongoing trials.

Side Effects of the Combined Therapy

The authors studying the effects of the combination of physostigmine and lecithin failed to report information regarding the side effects of the medications. Only Wettstein (1983) reported the presence of nausea and diarrhea in two of his eight patients; these side effects were described as mild.

Summers et al. (1986) reported several side effects in 17 patients receiving THA and lecithin. These side effects included nausea (in six patients), diaphoresis (in three), belching (in two), emesis (in three), abdominal discomfort (in three), diarrhea (in two), and increased micturition (in one). These patients were receiving 25–200 mg of THA in addition to orally administered lecithin for a period of 7–10 days. Gauthier et al. (1988) also used THA in combination with lecithin and reported several side effects (e.g., gastrointestinal disturbances). These side effects seemed to be dose-dependent and subsided with reduction of the dose of THA or with the administration of glycopyrrolate. In the more recent multicenter study reported above, Gauthier et al. (1990) reported side effects of the autonomic nervous system in 48% of the patients in the titration phase and 38% of the patients in the double-blind phase. These side effects were abdominal cramps (38%), nausea (25%), pollakiuria (25%) and, less frequently reported, diarrhea (23%), vomiting (18%), dizziness (19%), ptyalism (10%), palpitation (2%), reversible elevation of liver enzymes (17%), and a simple case of focal liver cell neurosis.

The available data on the use of anticholinesterase alone and in combination with lecithin or choline are not sufficient to draw a conclusion about the superiority of one drug over the combination of the drugs. However, this is an important area for further research.

Muscarinic Agonists

Both precursor loading (i.e., presynaptic drugs) and cholinesterase inhibition (i.e., synaptic drugs) are limited in that they require functional cholinergic neurons for drug activity. Several studies suggest that muscarinic agonists have the advantage of acting independently of presynaptic cholinergic neurons. The substitution of acetylcholine and the stimulation of postsynaptic cholinergic receptors may be effective in increasing central cholinergic functions. Postsynaptic cholinergic receptors are relatively intact in DAT. Preclinical studies also have demonstrated that cholinergic agonists are effective in enhancing performance in normal rodents and hypocholinergic animals in experimental situations (Davidson et al. 1988).

Recently, several cholinergic muscarinic agonists have been tested in DAT patients (Table 6-4). The main drugs are RS-86 (2-ethyl-8-methyl-2,8-diazospiro[4,5]-decase-1,3-dione hypobromide), bethanechol chloride, and arecoline. The latter drug has been reported to improve memory in some patients with DAT. However, arecoline's short duration of action, its rapid destruction by acetylcholinesterase, and the high incidence of adverse reactions have limited its use. The drug RS-86 is a potent muscarinic (mixed M_1-M_2 receptor) agonist with a relatively prolonged duration of central action following oral administration. It has analgesic and sedative properties in animals. In order to control many of the pharmacokinetic variables and to avoid the development of severe side effects, several researchers administered bethanechol chloride, a muscarinic agonist, directly into the cerebrospinal fluid (CSF). Intracerebral infusion pumps have been implanted with catheters running from the abdomen to the cerebral ventricles. Bethanechol does not cross the blood-brain barrier easily and is not destroyed by cholinesterases.

Besides the high incidence of side effects and the risks associated with surgery, the potential benefit of cholinergic agonists may be limited by their tonic action on the postsynaptic receptors. This effect is not similar to the physiologic phasic events of the cholinergic neurons (Hollander et al. 1987).

Efficacy

RS-86. Hollander et al. (1987) orally administered RS-86 to 12 patients (4 men and 8 women), aged 55–78 years, with DAT in a double-blind crossover study. RS-86 was found to improve both the cognitive and the noncognitive functions in 7 patients as measured by the Alzheimer's Disease Assesment Scale (ADAS) (Rosen et al. 1984). However, only 2 patients showed obvious clinical improvement.

Davidson et al. (1988) studied the effect of RS-86 on 15 patients aged 54–78 who met the NINCPS-ADRDA criteria of probable DAT.

Table 6–4. Effects of muscarinic agonists in patients with dementia of the Alzheimer type

Author (year)	Study	Number of patients	Age (years)	Dosage and method of administration	Duration	Effect on memory	Side effects
Bethanechol compounds							
Harbaugh et al. (1984)	Open clinical trial	4	64–73	0.05–0.7 mg/day ivi	8 months	++	Transient nausea, Parkinson's disease, sterile inflammatory response of CSF
Davous and Lamour (1985)	Double-blind clinical design	16	Mean = 65.4 ± 3.9 to 69.1 ± 2.3	0.25 mg methscopolamine + 0.1 mg/kg bethanechol sc	1 day	+	Abdominal cramps
Penn et al. (1988)	**Study 1:** Double-blind crossover	11	Mean = 64.9 ± 7.7	0.35 mg/day	24 weeks	0	Transient nausea
	Study 2: *Phase 1:* Double-blind crossover	9		0.35 mg→ 1.75 mg/day	8 weeks	0	Nausea, hyperventilation, myoclonus
	Phase 2: Open evaluating dose trial	8		0.35 mg→ 1.75 mg/day ivi	2 years	0	NR
Read (1988)	Open clinical trial	5	53–64	0.2–0.95 mg/day ivi	8–14 weeks	++	Agitation, dysphoria, depression, seizures, serious surgical morbidity (infection and hematoma)

RS-86

Study	Design	N	Age	Dose	Duration	Improvement	Adverse effects
Wettstein and Spiegel (1984)	Placebo-controlled dose-finding studies	17	65–90	3 mg orally	6 weeks	+	Nausea, dizziness; angina pectoris; general malaise; increased sweating and salivation; bronchospasm
Bruno et al. (1986)	Double-blind	8	Mean = 62 ±1.5 (55–68)	0.5 mg/day orally, increased gradually until 5 mg/day x 8 days orally	8 days	0	Diaphoresis, hypersalivation
Hollander et al. (1987)	Double-blind crossover	12	Mean = 66.1 (55–78)	0.5–1.5 mg tid x 7 days orally	2 weeks	+	Chills, tremors, crying spells, diaphoresis, hypersalivation, agitation, depression, syncope, abdominal distress, prolonged P-R interval
Davidson et al. (1988)	*Phase 1:* Open dose-finding study *Phase 2:* Double-blind crossover	15	54–78	1.5–4.5 mg/day x 7 days orally	3 weeks	+	Syncope, abdominal distress, seizures, chills, excessive sweating, flushing, depression, prolonged P-R interval, tremor, hypersalivation, confusion

Note. 0 = No improvement; + = mild improvement; ++ = moderate improvement; +++ = marked improvement; ivi = intraventricular infusion; CSF = cerebrospinal fluid; sc = subcutaneously.

All patients had a memory and information test score of 10 or less, a dementia rating score of 4 or more, and a Hachinski Ischemic Scale score of 5 or less. Patients received between 1.5 and 4.5 mg of RS-86. Examination of the performance on the ADAS subscales revealed no substantial RS-86 effect. Despite the lack of any effect on mean scores, 7 of 12 patients showed improvement on the overall ADAS scores in the replication phase. Three patients could not tolerate RS-86 and dropped out of the study. The less severe patients showed the most improvement.

Bruno et al. (1986) studied the effects of RS-86 on eight patients in a double-blind, placebo-controlled trial. Patients ranged from having mild to moderately advanced DAT. Testing showed some alterations on verbal and visuospatial tests, but no consistent overall change in cognitive performance was demonstrated.Wettstein and Spiegel (1984) gave 3 mg of RS-86 in a double-blind study over a period of 6 weeks. Positive clinical changes in cognitive functions, mood, and social behavior were seen in a minority of the DAT patients.

Bethanechol.　Penn et al. (1988) gave bethanechol by intraventricular infusion over a 24-week period in a double-blind crossover trial. Seven men and four women with a mean age of 64.9 years (and 3.9 years of dementia) were studied. The authors did not find any significant group differences in test scores either in the activities of daily living or in the objective cognitive measures. However, a moderate increase of the dosage (to 1.05 mg/day) may have had a palliative effect on patient behavior. Read (1988) gave bethanechol infusion to five patients with presenile onset dementia. Two patients experienced very severe medical and psychiatric complications. The other three patients maintained mild improvement for a period of 2 years. Harbaugh et al. (1984) gave bethanechol to four DAT patients in doses of 0.05 to 0.7 mg intracerebrally. All subjects showed improvement in cognitive and social functioning during drug infusion but returned to baseline performance with saline infusion. Davous and Lamour (1985) gave 0.1 mg bethanechol subcutaneously to eight patients with DAT. A significant shortening of reaction time was noticed in 15 minutes, but not 30 minutes, after the injection. In summary, bethanechol does not seem to have a promising future as a therapeutic agent for treatment of DAT.

Other muscarinic agonists.　Other muscarinic agonists, including arecoline and oxotremorine, have also been used in DAT patients.

Arecoline (4 mg) given intravenously was associated with only slight improvement. Oxotremorine (0.25–2.0 mg), another muscarinic agonist, was tried, but the severe side effects, particularly depression, made the continuation of these studies impossible (Davidson et al. 1988).

Side Effects

Oxotremorine was found to have significant adverse effects, making it difficult to evaluate its efficacy. Depressive symptoms occurred 1–5 hours after administration of higher doses. Oxotremorine stimulates receptors in a prolonged and tonic manner, which may be related to the severe depressive side effects of this drug.

Bethanechol was found to cause systemic side effects even when given through intraventricular infusion. The main side effects included nausea, abdominal cramps, Parkinson's disease (Harbaugh et al. 1984), myoclonus (Penn et al. 1988), agitation, dysphoria, and seizures (Read 1988). Furthermore, intraventricular catheterization also carries several surgical risks such as infection, stroke, and intracranial bleeding.

RS-86 was found to cause nausea, malaise, autonomic side effects, dizziness, salivation bronchospasm, diaphoresis, chills and confusion, seizures, and a prolonged P-R interval.

Future Considerations

We have known about the existence of cholinergic deficits in DAT patients for more than a decade now, and several attempts have been made to correct these deficits. However, the results are not very encouraging. The severe side effects associated with various drugs in this group have hampered the progress in correcting cholinergic deficits. We need to develop drugs with a longer duration of action and fewer side effects. These new drugs should enhance cholinergic activity and possibly have an effect on other neurotransmitter and neuromodulation systems. It appears that DAT patients have deficits of several neurotransmitters and neuromodulators and thus require a multifaceted approach.

However, ethical problems associated with new experimental treatment in DAT patients should not be overlooked. Unfortunately, as evident from the review, most of these treatments showing some promise have a considerable degree of unpleasant and potentially serious side effects. Because DAT patients cannot always give an informed consent, we must take precautions while using unproven treatments.

References

Agnoli A, Martucci N, Manna V, et al: Effect of cholinergic and anticholinergic drugs on short-term memory in Alzheimer's dementia: a neuropsychologic and computerized electroencephalographic study. Clin Neuropharmacol 6:311–323, 1983

Ames PJ, Bhathal PS, Davies BM, et al: Hepatotoxicity of tetrahydroaminoacridine (letter). Lancet 1:887, 1988

Bajada S: A trial of choline chloride and physostigmine in Alzheimer's dementia, in Alzheimer's Disease: A Report of Progress (Aging, Vol 19). Edited by Corkin S, Davis KL, Growdon JW, et al. New York, Raven, pp 427–432, 1982

Becker RE, Elble R, Kumar V, et al: Effects of metrifonate, a long-acting cholinesterase inhibitor in Alzheimer disease: report of an open trial. Drug Developmental Research (in press)

Beller SA, Overall JE, Swann AC: Efficacy of oral physostigmine in primary degenerative dementia: a double-blind study of response to different dose levels. Psychopharmacology (Berlin) 87:147–151, 1985

Beller SA, Overall JE, Rhoades HM, et al: Long-term outpatient treatment of senile dementia with oral physostigmine. J Clin Psychiatry 49(10):400–404, 1988

Blackwood D, Christie JE: The effects of physostigmine on memory and auditory P300 in Alzheimer-type dementia. Biol Psychiatry 21:557–560, 1986

Boyd WD, Graham-White J, Blackwood G, et al: Clinical effects of choline in Alzheimer senile dementia. Lancet 2:711, 1977

Brinkman SD, Pomara N, Goodnick PJ, et al: A dose-ranging study of lecithin in the treatment of primary degenerative dementia (Alzheimer disease). J Clin Psychopharmacology 2:281–285, 1982

Bruno G, Mohr E, Gillespie M, et al: Muscarinic agonist therapy of Alzheimer's disease: a clinical trial of RS-86. Arch Neurol 43:659–661, 1986

Caltagirone C, Gainotti G, Masullo C: Oral administration of chronic physostigmine does not improve cognitive or amnesic performances in Alzheimer's presenile dementia. Int J Neurosci 16:247–249, 1982

Christie JE, Shering A, Ferguson J, et al: Physostigmine and arecoline: effects of intravenous infusions in Alzheimer presenile dementia. Br J Psychiatry 138:46–50, 1981

Cohen EL, Wurtman RJ: Brain acetylcholine: increase after systemic choline administration. Life Sci 16:1095–1102, 1975

Cohen E, Wurtman R: Brain acetylcholine: control by dietary intake. Science 191:561–562, 1976

Coyle JT, Price PI, DeLong MR: Alzheimer's disease: a disorder of cortical cholinergic innervation. Science 219:1184–1190, 1983

Davidson M, Hollander E, Zemishlany Z, et al: Cholinergic agonists in Alzheimer's disease patients, in Current Research in Alzheimer's Therapy. Edited by Giacobini E, Becker RE. New York, Taylor & Francis, 1988, pp 333–336

Davies P, Maloney AJF: Selective loss of central cholinergic neurons in Alzheimer's disease. Lancet 2:1403, 1976

Davis KL, Mohs RC: Enhancement of memory process in Alzheimer's disease with multiple-dose intravenous physostigmine. Am J Psychiatry 139:1421–1424, 1982

Davis KL, Mohs RC, Tinklenberg JR: Enhancement of memory by physostigmine. N Engl J Med 301:946, 1979

Davous P, Lamour Y: Bethanechol decreases reaction time in senile dementia of the Alzheimer type. J Neurol Neurosurg Psychiatry 48:1297–1299, 1985

Domino EF, Louise M, Puff IF, et al: Effects of oral lecithin on blood choline levels and memory tests in geriatric volunteers, in Alzheimer's Disease: A Report of Progress (Aging, Vol 19). Edited by Corkin S, Davis KL, Growdon JW, et al. New York, Raven, 1982, pp 393–398

Dysken MW, Fovall P, Harris CM, et al: Lecithin administration in Alzheimer dementia. Neurology 32:1202–1203, 1982a

Dysken MW, Fovall P, Harris CM, et al: Lecithin administration in patients with primary degenerative dementia and in normal volunteers, in Alzheimer's Disease: A Report of Progress (Aging, Vol 19). Edited by Corkin S, Davis KL, Growdon JW, et al. New York, Raven, 1982b, pp 385–392

Elble RJ, Giacobini E, Becker RE, et al: Treatment of Alzheimer dementia with steady-state infusion of physostigmine, in Current Research in Alzheimer's Therapy. Edited by Giacobini E, Becker RE. New York, Taylor & Francis, 1988, pp 403–407

Etienne P, Gauthier S, Dastoor P, et al: Lecithin in Alzheimer's disease. Lancet 2:1206, 1978a

Etienne P, Gauthier S, Johnson G, et al: Clinical effects of choline in Alzheimer's disease. Lancet 1:508–509, 1978b

Ferris SH, Reisberg O, Crook T, et al: Pharmacologic treatment of senile dementia: choline, L-DOPA, piracetam, and choline plus piracetam, in Alzheimer's Disease: A Report of Progress (Aging, Vol 19). Edited by Corkin S, Davis KL, Growdon JW, et al. New York, Raven, 1982, pp 475–481

Fitten LJ, Perryman KM, Gross PL, et al: Chronic oral THA administration in mice, monkeys, and man. Paper presented at the International Symposium on Advances in Alzheimer Therapy, Springfield, IL, 1988

Fitten LJ, Perryman KM, Gross PL, et al: Treatment of Alzheimer's disease with short- and long-term oral THA and lecithin: a double-blind study. Am J Psychiatry 147:239–242, 1990

Fovall P, Dysken MW, Lazarus LW, et al: Choline bitartrate treatment of Alzheimer's type dementia. Communication in Psychopharmacology 4:141–145, 1980

Gauthier S, Masson H, Gauthier L, et al: Tetrahydroaminoacridine and lecithin in Alzheimer's disease, in Current Research in Alzheimer's Therapy. Edited by Giacobini E, Becker RE. New York, Taylor & Francis, 1988, pp 237–245

Gauthier S, Bouchard R, Lawontagne A, et al: Tetrahydroaminoacridine-lecithin combination treatment in patients with intermediate-stage Alzheimer's disease. N Engl J Med 322:1272–1276, 1990

Glen AIM, Yates CM, Simpson J, et al: Choline uptake in patients with Alzheimer pre-senile dementia. Psychol Med 11:469–476, 1981

Harbaugh RE, Roberts DW, Coombs PW, et al: Preliminary report: intracranial cholinergic drug infusion in patients with Alzheimer's disease. Neurosurgery 15:514–518, 1984

Haubrich DR, Chippendale TJ: Regulation of acetylcholine synthesis in nervous tissue. Life Sci 20:1465–1478, 1977

Heyman A, Logue P, Wilkinson W, et al: Lecithin therapy of Alzheimer's disease: a preliminary report, in Alzheimer's Disease: A Report of Progress (Aging, Vol 19). Edited by Corkin S, Davis KL, Growdon JW, et al. New York, Raven, 1982, pp 373–383

Hollander E, Davidson M, Mohs RC, et al: RS-86 in the treatment of Alzheimer's disease: cognitive and biological effects. Biol Psychiatry 22:1067–1078, 1987

Jenike MA, Albert MS, Heller H, et al: Combination therapy with lecithin and ergoloid mesylates for Alzheimer's disease. J Clin Psychiatry 47(5):249–251, 1986

Johns CA, Haroutunian V, Greenwald BS, et al: Development of cholinergic drugs for the treatment of Alzheimer's disease. Drug Developmental Research 5:77–96, 1985

Jotkowitz S: Lack of clinical efficacy of chronic oral physostigmine in Alzheimer's disease. Ann Neurol 14:690–691, 1983

Kaye WH, Sitaram N, Weingartner H, et al: Modest facilitation of memory in dementia with combined lecithin and anticholinesterase treatment. Biol Psychiatry 17:275–280, 1982

Kumar V: Efficacy and side effects of THA in Alzheimer's disease patients, in Current Research in Alzheimer's Therapy. Edited by Giacobini E, Becker RE. New York, Taylor & Francis, 1988, pp 225–229

Kumar V, Becker RE: Clinical pharmacology of tetrahydroaminoacridine: a possible therapeutic agent for Alzheimer's disease. Int J Clin Pharmacol Ther Toxicol 27:478–485, 1989

Levy R: Cholinergic side effects of tetrahydroaminoacridine (letter). Lancet 2:1421, 1988

Little A, Levy R, Chuaqui-Kidd P, et al: A double-blind, placebo-controlled trial of high-dose lecithin in Alzheimer's disease. J Neurol Neurosurg Psychiatry 48:736–742, 1985

Mayeux R, Albert M, Jenike M: Physostigmine-induced myoclonus in Alzheimer's disease. Neurology 37:345–346, 1987

Mohs RC, Davis KL, Tinklenberg JR, et al: Choline chloride treatment of memory deficits in the elderly. Am J Psychiatry 136:1275–1277, 1979

Mohs RC, Davis BM, Johns CA, et al: Oral physostigmine treatment of patients with Alzheimer's disease. Am J Psychiatry 142:28–33, 1985

Muramoto O, Sugishita M, Sugita H, et al: Effect of physostigmine on constructional and memory tasks in Alzheimer's disease. Arch Neurol 36:501–503, 1979

Muramoto O, Sugishita M, Ando K: Cholinergic system and constructional praxis: a further study of physostigmine in Alzheimer's disease. J Neurol Neurosurg Psychiatry 47:485–491, 1984

Nyback H, Nyman H, Ohman G, et al: Preliminary experiences with THA for the amelioration of symptoms of Alzheimer's disease, in Current Research in Alzheimer's Therapy. Edited by Giacobini E, Becker RE. New York, Taylor & Francis, 1988, pp 231–236

Penn RD, Wilson RS, Fox JH, et al: Intraventricular bethanechol for Alzheimer's disease: results of double-blind and escalating dose trials, in Current Research in Alzheimer's Therapy. Edited by Giacobini E, Becker RE. New York, Taylor & Francis, 1988, pp 325–331

Perry EK, Perry RH, Blessed G, et al: Necropsy evidence of central cholinergic deficits in senile dementia. Lancet 1:189, 1977

Peters BH, Levin HS: Effects of physostigmine and lecithin on memory in Alzheimer disease. Ann Neurol 6:219–221, 1979

Peters BH, Levin HS: Chronic oral physostigmine and lecithin administration in memory disorders of aging, in Alzheimer's Disease: A Report of Progress (Aging, Vol 19). Edited by Corkin S, Davis KL, Growdon JW, et al. New York, Raven, 1982, pp 421–426

Pomara N, Domino EF, Yoon H, et al: Failure of single-dose lecithin to alter aspects of central cholinergic activity in Alzheimer's disease. J Clin Psychiatry 44(8):293–295, 1983

Read S: Intra-cerebro-ventricular bethanechol: dose and response, in Current Research in Alzheimer's Therapy. Edited by Giacobini E, Becker RE. New York, Taylor & Francis, 1988, pp 315–324

Renvoize EB, Jerram T: Choline in Alzheimer's disease. N Engl J Med 301:330, 1979

Rose RP, Moulthrop MA: Differential responsivity of verbal and visual recognition memory to physostigmine and ACTH. Biol Psychiatry 21:538–542, 1986

Rosen WG, Mohs RC, Davis KL: A new rating scale for Alzheimer's disease. Am J Psychiatry 141:1356–1364, 1983

Rossor MN, Iversen LL, Reynolds GP, et al: Neurochemical characteristics of early and late onset types of Alzheimer's disease. Br Med J 288:961–964, 1984

Roth M, Wischik CM: Heterogeneity of Alzheimer's disease and its implications for scientific investigations of the disorder, in Recent Advances in Psychogeriatrics. Edited by Aire T. Edinburgh, Churchill Livingstone, 1985, pp 71–92

Schwartz AS, Kohlstaedt EV: Physostigmine effects in Alzheimer's disease: relationship to dementia severity. Life Sci 38:1021–1028, 1986

Signoret JL, Whiteley A, Lhermitte F: Influence of choline on amnesia in early Alzheimer's disease. Lancet 2:837, 1978

Sims NR, Bowen PM, Allen SJ, et al: Presynaptic cholinergic dysfunction in patients with dementia. J Neurochem 40:503–509, 1983

Smith CM, Swash M: Physostigmine in Alzheimer's disease. Lancet 1:42, 1979

Smith CM, Swash M, Exton-Smith AN, et al: Choline therapy in Alzheimer's disease. Lancet 2:318, 1978

Smith CM, Semple SA, Swash M: Effects of physostigmine on responses in memory tests in patients with Alzheimer's disease, in Alzheimer's Disease: A Report of Progress (Aging, Vol 19). Edited by Corkin S, Davis KL, Growdon JW, et al. New York, Raven, 1982, pp 405–411

Stern Y, Sano M, Mayeux R: Long-term administration of oral physostigmine in Alzheimer's disease. Neurology 38:1837–1841, 1988

Sullivan EV, Shedlack KJ, Corkin S, et al: Physostigmine and lecithin in Alzheimer's disease, in Alzheimer's Disease: A Report of Progress (Aging, Vol 19). Edited by Corkin S, Davis KL, Growdon JW, et al. New York, Raven, 1982, pp 361–367

Summers WK, Viesselman JO, Marsh GM, et al: Use of THA in treatment of Alzheimer-like dementia: pilot study in twelve patients. Biol Psychiatry 16:145–153, 1981

Summers WK, Majovski LV, Marsh GM, et al: Oral tetrahydroaminoacridine in long-term treatment of senile dementia, Alzheimer type. N Engl J Med 315:1241–1245, 1986

Thal LJ, Fuld PA: Memory enhancement with oral physostigmine in Alzheimer's disease. N Engl J Med 308:720, 1983

Thal LJ, Fuld PA, Mazur DM, et al: Oral physostigmine and lecithin improve memory in Alzheimer's disease. Ann Neurol 13:491–496, 1983

Thal LJ, Masur DM, Sharpless NS, et al: Acute and chronic effects of oral physostigmine and lecithin in Alzheimer's disease. Prog Neuropsychopharmacol Biol Psychiatry 10:627–636, 1986

Thal LJ, Masur DM, Blau AD, et al: Chronic oral physostigmine without lecithin improves memory in Alzheimer's disease. J Am Geriatr Soc 37:42–48, 1989

Vroulis GA, Smith RC, Brinkman S, et al: The effects of lecithin on memory in patients with senile dementia of the Alzheimer's type. Psychopharmacol Bull 17:127–128, 1981

Weintraub S, Mesulam M-M, Auty R, et al: Lecithin in the treatment of Alzheimer's disease. Arch Neurol 40:527–528, 1983

Wettstein A: No effect from double-blind trial of physostigmine and lecithin in Alzheimer disease. Arch Neurol 13:210–212, 1983

Wettstein A, Spiegel R: Clinical trials with the cholinergic drug RS-86 in Alzheimer's disease (AD) and senile dementia of the Alzheimer type (SDAT). Psychopharmacology (Berlin) 84:572–573, 1984

Whelpton R: Analysis of plasma physostigmine concentrations by liquid chromatography. J Chromatogr 272:216–220, 1981

Whitehouse PJ, Price DL, Struble RG, et al: Alzheimer's disease and senile dementia: loss of neurons in the basal forebrain. Science 125:1237–1239, 1982

Wilcock GK, Surmon D, Forsyth D, et al: Cholinergic side effects of tetrahydroaminoacridine (letter). Lancet 2:1305, 1988

Wood JL, Allison RG: Effects of consumption of choline and lecithin on neurological and cardiovascular systems. Federation Proceedings 41:3015–3016, 1982

Wurtman RJ, Hirsch MJ, Growdon JH: Lecithin consumption raises serum-free-choline levels. Lancet 2:68–69, 1977

Index